PHYSICS IN RADIATION ONCOLOGY
SELF-ASSESSMENT GUIDE

PHYSICS IN RADIATION ONCOLOGY
SELF-ASSESSMENT GUIDE

Edited by

Andrew Godley, PhD
Staff Physicist
Department of Radiation Oncology
Taussig Cancer Institute
Cleveland Clinic
Cleveland, Ohio

Ping Xia, PhD
Head of Medical Physics
Professor of Molecular Medicine
Department of Radiation Oncology
Taussig Cancer Institute
Cleveland Clinic
Cleveland, Ohio

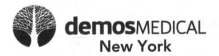

demosMEDICAL
New York

Visit our website at www.demosmedical.com

ISBN: 9781620700709
e-book ISBN: 9781617052408

Acquisitions Editor: Rich Winters
Compositor: diacriTech

Medicine is an ever-changing science. Research and clinical experience are continually expanding our knowledge, in particular our understanding of proper treatment and drug therapy. The authors, editors, and publisher have made every effort to ensure that all information in this book is in accordance with the state of knowledge at the time of production of the book. Nevertheless, the authors, editors, and publisher are not responsible for errors or omissions or for any consequences from application of the information in this book and make no warranty, expressed or implied, with respect to the contents of the publication. Every reader should examine carefully the package inserts accompanying each drug and should carefully check whether the dosage schedules mentioned therein or the contraindications stated by the manufacturer differ from the statements made in this book. Such examination is particularly important with drugs that are either rarely used or have been newly released on the market.

Library of Congress Cataloging-in-Publication Data

Physics in radiation oncology : self-assessment guide / editors, Andrew Godley, Ping Xia.
    p. ; cm.
  Includes bibliographical references and index.
  ISBN 978-1-62070-070-9
  I. Godley, Andrew, editor. II. Xia, Ping (Radiation oncologist), editor.
  [DNLM: 1. Health Physics—methods—Examination Questions. 2. Neoplasms—radiotherapy—Examination Questions. QZ 18.2]
  RC271.R3
  616.99'40642076—dc23
                        2015015028

Special discounts on bulk quantities of Demos Medical Publishing books are available to corporations, professional associations, pharmaceutical companies, health care organizations, and other qualifying groups. For details, please contact:

Special Sales Department
Demos Medical Publishing, LLC
11 West 42nd Street, 15th Floor
New York, NY 10036
Phone: 800-532-8663 or 212-683-0072
Fax: 212-941-7842
E-mail: specialsales@demosmedical.com

Printed in the United States of America by Gasch.
15 16 17 18 / 5 4 3 2 1

CONTENTS

Contents

CONTRIBUTORS

Martin Andrews, PhD
Department of Radiation Oncology
Taussig Cancer Institute
Cleveland Clinic
Cleveland, Ohio

Salim Balik, PhD
Department of Radiation Oncology
Taussig Cancer Institute
Cleveland Clinic
Cleveland, Ohio

Henry Blair, MD
Department of Radiation Oncology
Taussig Cancer Institute
Cleveland Clinic
Cleveland, Ohio

Toufik Djemil, PhD
Department of Radiation Oncology
Taussig Cancer Institute
Cleveland Clinic
Cleveland, Ohio

Frank Dong, PhD
Diagnostic Radiology
Imaging Institute
Cleveland Clinic
Cleveland, Ohio

Andrew Godley, PhD
Department of Radiation Oncology
Taussig Cancer Institute
Cleveland Clinic
Cleveland, Ohio

Jeff Kittel, MD
Department of Radiation Oncology
Taussig Cancer Institute
Cleveland Clinic
Cleveland, Ohio

Matthew Kolar, MS
Department of Radiation Oncology
Taussig Cancer Institute
Cleveland Clinic
Cleveland, Ohio

Anthony Magnelli, MS
Department of Radiation Oncology
Taussig Cancer Institute
Cleveland Clinic
Cleveland, Ohio

Anthony Mastroianni, MD
Department of Radiation Oncology
Taussig Cancer Institute
Cleveland Clinic
Cleveland, Ohio

Diana Mattson, CMD
Department of Radiation Oncology
Taussig Cancer Institute
Cleveland Clinic
Cleveland, Ohio

Lama Muhieddine Mossolly, MS
Department of Radiation Oncology
Taussig Cancer Institute
Cleveland Clinic
Cleveland, Ohio

Mihir Naik, DO
Department of Radiation Oncology
Taussig Cancer Institute
Cleveland Clinic
Cleveland, Ohio

Gennady Neyman, PhD
Department of Radiation Oncology
Taussig Cancer Institute
Cleveland Clinic
Cleveland, Ohio

Yvonne Pham, MD
Department of Radiation Oncology
Taussig Cancer Institute
Cleveland Clinic
Cleveland, Ohio

Peng Qi, PhD
Department of Radiation Oncology
Taussig Cancer Institute
Cleveland Clinic
Cleveland, Ohio

Maria Rybak, MS
Department of Radiation Oncology
Taussig Cancer Institute
Cleveland Clinic
Cleveland, Ohio

Qingyang Shang, PhD
Department of Radiation Oncology
Taussig Cancer Institute
Cleveland Clinic
Cleveland, Ohio

Zhilei Liu Shen, PhD
Department of Radiation Oncology
Taussig Cancer Institute
Cleveland Clinic
Cleveland, Ohio

Nicholas Shkumat, MS
Diagnostic Radiology
Imaging Institute
Cleveland Clinic
Cleveland, Ohio

Mike Strongosky, MS
Department of Radiation Oncology
Taussig Cancer Institute
Cleveland Clinic
Cleveland, Ohio

Eric Tischler, MS
Department of Radiation Oncology
Taussig Cancer Institute
Cleveland Clinic
Cleveland, Ohio

Matthew Vossler, MS
Department of Radiation Oncology
Taussig Cancer Institute
Cleveland Clinic
Cleveland, Ohio

Matthew C. Ward, MD
Department of Radiation Oncology
Taussig Cancer Institute
Cleveland Clinic
Cleveland, Ohio

Allan Wilkinson, PhD
Department of Radiation Oncology
Taussig Cancer Institute
Cleveland Clinic
Cleveland, Ohio

Neil Woody, MD
Department of Radiation Oncology
Taussig Cancer Institute
Cleveland Clinic
Cleveland, Ohio

Kevin Wunderle, MS
Diagnostic Radiology
Imaging Institute
Cleveland Clinic
Cleveland, Ohio

Naichang Yu, PhD
Department of Radiation Oncology
Taussig Cancer Institute
Cleveland Clinic
Cleveland, Ohio

Tingliang Zhuang, PhD
Department of Radiation Oncology
Taussig Cancer Institute
Cleveland Clinic
Cleveland, Ohio

Lisa Zickefoose, CMD
Department of Radiation Oncology
Taussig Cancer Institute
Cleveland Clinic
Cleveland, Ohio

PREFACE

We are delighted to introduce the first edition of the *Physics in Radiation Oncology Self-Assessment Guide*. This guide provides a comprehensive physics review for anyone in the Radiation Oncology field. It partners the 2013 release of the *Radiation Oncology Self-Assessment Guide*, enhancing the resources available to scholars of radiation oncology. This book was designed as a flash card, question and answer style to help reinforce concepts and provide a focused review of medical physics. The detailed answers allow the reader to learn through completing the questions. The topics covered are expansive and thorough, effectively covering the same range as a radiation oncology physics text.

The guide has been divided into 14 chapters, leading the reader through the radiation oncology physics field, from basic physics to current practice and latest innovations. Basic physics covers fundamentals, photon and particle interactions, and dose measurement. All of current practice is included; treatment planning, safety, regulations, quality assurance, and SBRT, SRS, TBI, IMRT, and IGRT techniques. A unique aspect of the guide is its chapter dedicated to the topics in diagnostic imaging most relevant to radiation oncology, covering MRI, ultrasound, fluoroscopy, mammography, PET, SPECT, and CT. New technologies, such as VMAT, novel IGRT devices, proton therapy, and MRI-guided therapy, are also incorporated.

This book has been written by the medical physicists in the Department of Radiation Oncology at the Cleveland Clinic Taussig Cancer Institute with help from the entire department including radiation oncology residents, dosimetrists, and staff physicians; and our physicist colleagues in the Imaging Institute at the Cleveland Clinic. It is our sincere wish that this guide becomes an excellent resource for anyone wishing to reinforce their knowledge of medical physics.

Andrew Godley, PhD
Ping Xia, PhD

PHYSICS IN RADIATION ONCOLOGY
SELF-ASSESSMENT GUIDE

1

FUNDAMENTAL PHYSICS

MIHIR NAIK AND ANDREW GODLEY

Question 1
What are the units of radioactivity?

Question 2
What is a roentgen (R) and what is it used for?

Question 3
What is the SI unit for absorbed dose?

Question 4
What is the relationship between Sievert (Sv) and rem?

Answer 1

The units of radioactivity are the Becquerel (Bq) and Curie (Ci). 1 Bq = 1 decay/sec. 1 curie = 3.7×10^{10} decay/sec, thus 1 mCi = 3.7×10^7 Bq.

Answer 2

A roentgen is the unit of exposure. Exposure is the measure of ionization of photon radiation in air, defined as the charge of one sign released per unit mass. 1R = 2.58×10^{-4} C/kg at standard temperature (0°C) and pressure (760 mmHg).

Answer 3

The SI unit for absorbed dose is the gray (Gy) such that 1 Gy = 1 J/kg. Rad is the former unit for absorbed dose, 1 Gy = 100 rad, and 1 rad = 1 cGy.

Answer 4

The Sv and rem measure the effect of dose on the body. It includes the biological effect of different types of radiation such as neutrons (equivalent dose), or the increased sensitivity of different organs (effective dose). The SI unit is the Sv. 1 Sv = 1 J/kg and 1 mSv = 100 mrem.

Question 5
What is the relationship between an atomic mass unit (amu) and an electron volt (eV)?

Question 6
How does a photon's energy relate to its frequency and wavelength?

Question 7
What is the electromagnetic spectrum?

Question 8
What is the SI unit of specific activity?

Answer 5

The electron volt is defined as the kinetic energy given to an electron initially at rest going through a potential difference of 1 V. It is a unit of energy with 1 eV = 1.602×10^{-19} Joules (J) and 1 amu = 931 MeV. The amu represents one twelfth of the mass of a carbon-12 nucleus.

Answer 6

The energy of a photon equals its frequency (in Hz) multiplied by Planck's constant ($h = 6.26 \times 10^{-34}$ J sec). Frequency (ν) is related to wavelength (λ) by $c = \lambda \nu$. The velocity (c) is the speed of light, 3×10^8 m/sec.

Answer 7

Photons travel as electromagnetic waves, described by the electromagnetic spectrum. This spectrum defines regions based on their energy (and hence wavelength or frequency). From lowest energy (and lowest frequency, highest wavelength) the spectrum starts with radio waves, then microwaves, infrared, visible, ultraviolet, X-rays, and gamma rays.

Answer 8

Specific activity is defined as a sample's activity (A) divided by its mass (m). The SI unit for specific activity is Bq/kg. It can also be given in terms of Ci/g. A higher specific activity allows a smaller source to be used for radiation treatment. For example, the specific activity of ^{60}Co source is 200 Ci/g and could contain 6,000 to 7,000 Ci in a 1.5 to 2.0 cm diameter ^{60}Co source.

Question 9
What is Planck's constant and how is it used to calculate the energy of a photon?

Question 10
What is the relationship between energy and wavelength and how can that relationship be used to calculate the energy of a photon?

Question 11
What is the Avogadro constant?

Question 1   **1.2 ATOMIC AND NUCLEAR STRUCTURE**
What is the charge of an electron?

Answer 9

Planck's constant (h) is given as $h = 6.62 \times 10^{-34}$ J sec. A photon does not possess any mass or have any charge, but does possess energy which is related to the frequency (v) of the photon by the following equation, $E = hv$.

Answer 10

We know that $c = v\lambda$, where λ is the wavelength and c is the speed of light (3×10^8 m/sec). By using this relationship, we can determine the frequency v and then use $E = hv$ to calculate the energy of a photon.

Answer 11

The Avogadro constant is $N_A = 6.022 \times 10^{23}$, which is the number of atoms in a mole of a substance.

Answer 1

The charge of an electron is 1.6×10^{-19} C. A Coulomb (C) is a unit of electric charge and represents a total charge of 6.24×10^{18} electrons. In classical physics, the smallest unit of negative charge is an electron with a charge of "−1" while the proton has the smallest unit of positive charge, "+1."

Question 2

What is the binding energy of an electron?

Question 3

What is the maximum number of electrons that can be placed in a shell?

Question 4

What is the charge and mass (MeV) of an electron, proton, and neutron?

Question 5

For an atom designated by the following atomic symbol: $_Z^A X$, how does one determine the atomic mass number, the number of protons, electrons, and neutrons in the atom as well as the number of nucleons?

Answer 2

The electron binding energy is determined by the Coulomb attraction between the nucleus (protons) and orbital electrons (e^-). The electron binding energy increases as Z increases and decreases as the distance from the nucleus increases. The binding energy of an electron is the minimum energy required to knock the electron out of the atom.

Answer 3

Electron shells are labeled starting from the inner most shell by letters or by numbers. The inner most shell is the "K Shell" followed by the L, M, and N shells, respectively. The maximum number of electrons that can be allowed in a shell is $2n^2$, where n is the shell number from the inner most to outer most orbital, ($K = 1$, $L = 2$). However, the outer most shell of an atom commonly referred to as the valance shell is only able to carry eight electrons.

Answer 4

An electron has a charge of -1 and a rest mass of 0.511 MeV. The mass of an electron is 1/1,836 compared to the mass of a proton. The proton has a charge of $+1$, and a rest mass of 938 MeV. The neutron has a charge of 0, and a rest mass of 939 MeV.

Answer 5

For a given atomic symbol, the number of protons is equal to "Z" which is also equal to the number of electrons. "A" is the mass number which is also equal to the number of protons + neutrons and is also referred to as the number of nucleons. The number of neutrons is equal to $A - Z$.

Question 6

Arrange the following forces (weak force, strong force, gravitational force, and electromagnetic force) in order from weakest to strongest and describe their basic responsibilities.

Question 7

What is an isotope, isotone, isobar, and isomer?

Question 8

What is a characteristic X-ray?

Question 9

What is an Auger electron?

Answer 6

The weakest is the gravitational force which is the force that attracts masses, but on the scale of the atomic world it is negligible. Next, the weak force is responsible for nuclear decay. The electromagnetic force exists between all particles which have an electric charge. The strong force is responsible for binding nuclei and exists over a very short range.

Answer 7

An element is defined by its atomic number Z, which represents the number of protons, and gives the element its *chemical* properties. The same element can have differing numbers of neutrons but the same number of protons, these are referred to as isotopes. An isotone is the opposite, they are nuclei with the same number of neutrons, but different numbers of protons. Isobars are nuclei that have the same number of nucleons (eg, seven protons and eight neutrons, or six protons and nine neutrons), that is the same atomic number. A helpful guide is istoPes have equal number of Protons, isotoNes have equal Neutrons, and isobArs have same atomic weight (A). An isomer is the same nucleus (the same number of protons, neutrons, and the same atomic number) but is an excited, usually unstable state of the nucleus.

Answer 8

If an atom is ionized, a vacancy may be created in an inner electron orbital. An electron in an outer orbital will then fill the vacancy and a photon with energy equal to the difference in energy of the two orbitals is created. This energy is characteristic of the particular element involved (hence the name).

Answer 9

An Auger electron is an alternative and competing process to characteristic X-rays that can sometimes occur. Here, instead of a characteristic X-ray escaping the atom, it hits another orbiting electron, which is ejected from the atom. This is known as an Auger electron.

Question 10
What is the difference between fission and fusion?

Question 11
Why do fission and fusion occur?

Question 12
What is the fluorescent yield?

Question 13
What is the difference between an X-ray and a gamma ray?

Answer 10

Fission is the splitting of a large unstable nucleus into more stable pieces. Fusion combines two or more lighter nuclei into one, as occurs in the sun when hydrogen is fused to form helium.

Answer 11

The binding energy per nucleon has a maximum near $A = 56$, and the average binding energy (except for light elements) is about 8 MeV per nucleon. Both fission (for $A > 56$) and fusion (for $A < 56$) occur to enable nuclei to approach a more stable state that is closer to the maximum binding energy per nucleon.

Answer 12

The fluorescent yield ω is defined as the probability that an atom will yield characteristic radiation rather than an Auger electron. The following relationships are noted:
High-Z → large ω → emission of characteristic radiation more probable
Low-Z → small ω → emission of Auger electrons more probable.

Answer 13

X-rays and gamma rays are both photons and forms of electromagnetic energy but gamma rays are defined as being of nuclear origin, and X-rays of atomic origin.

Question 14
What are the two competing mechanisms by which the nucleus can release excess energy in isomeric transition?

Question 1   1.3 RADIOACTIVITY
How is the decay constant of a nucleus related to its half-life?

Question 2
Describe the type of equilibrium that can occur with radioactive decay when the decay constant of the daughter is much greater than the parent decay constant?

Question 3
What are the two types of decay that tend to occur in nuclei that have a low neutron to proton (n/p) ratio?

Answer 14

An isomeric transition means the nucleus is changing energy states, without changing the number of protons and neutrons within it. One way the nucleus can release energy is called gamma emission. In gamma emission, the nucleus releases excess energy by the direct emission of one or more gamma rays from the nucleus. An alternative method of releasing energy is internal conversion where one or more of the orbital electrons is emitted. If an inner shell electron is emitted, shell filling will occur and will result in characteristic X-rays and/or Auger electrons being released.

Answer 1

The decay constant is related to the half-life: $\lambda = \ln(2)/T_{1/2}$

Answer 2

This type of equilibrium is called secular equilibrium. This is characterized by a gradual buildup of activity of the daughter until it reaches the level of the parent. After secular equilibrium has been established, the activity of the daughter is approximately equal to the activity of the parent. This is the case for Radium and its daughter Radon. The decay constant is inversely proportional to the half-life, so for secular equilibrium, the daughter half-life must be much shorter than the parent. If the decay constant of the daughter is greater than the decay constant of the parent but not much greater, then transient equilibrium is achieved. In transient equilibrium, there is an initial buildup of the daughter until it eventually exceeds the activity of the parent. After that point, the activity of the daughter follows the activity of the parent, always exceeding the parent by a small amount. This is exemplified by Mo-99 (molybdenum) and its daughter Tc-99m (Technetium).

Answer 3

Radionuclides that have a low n/p ratio tend to increase the ratio by converting a proton into a neutron. In beta plus decay or positron emission, the proton converts into a neutron emitting a positive electron (positron or beta plus) and a neutrino.

A competing process with beta plus decay is electron capture. Here, one of the inner orbital electrons (usually K shell) is captured by the nucleus. The nucleus rearranges and transforms a proton into a neutron to reach a new stable state. After an electron is captured by the nucleus in electron capture decay, characteristic X-rays or Auger electrons will be produced.

Question 4
Describe the differences in the neutron to proton ratio (n/p) with respect to the atomic number of the nucleus?

Question 5
What is isomeric transition?

Question 6
What is isobaric decay?

Question 7
What is the nuclear binding energy?

Answer 4

For atomic elements where Z is less than or equal to 20, the ratio of neutrons to protons is 1. If Z is greater than 20, the ratio increases with Z. The additional neutrons are needed to help keep the nuclei stable and to compensate for electrostatic repulsion between the protons.

Answer 5

Isomeric transition occurs when a previous radioactive decay leaves the daughter nucleus in a metastable state which then transitions to the ground state. The daughter nucleus stays in an excited state for a short period of time. The only difference between the metastable state and the final stable ground state is an energy difference, thus the two states are called isomers. An example of this is technetium-99m. Molybdenum-99 decays via beta decay to Tc-99m. In this metastable state, it has a half-life of 6 hours. It then decays via gamma emission, releasing a photon of 141 keV, which is used for imaging in single-photon emission computed tomography (SPECT).

Answer 6

Isobaric decay is any radioactive decay in which the original (or parent) nucleus and the new (or daughter) nucleus contains the same number of total nucleons (protons + neutrons). When this occurs, the parent nucleus and the daughter nucleus are referred to as isobars of one another. Both types of beta decay are isobaric.

Answer 7

The nucleus is made up of protons and neutrons, but the mass of the nucleus will always be less than the sum of the individual masses of the protons and neutrons which constitute it. The deficiency of mass is called the mass defect, and the energy that is required to separate the nucleus into its constituent particles is called the binding energy of the nucleus and is given by Einstein's famous equation: $E = \Delta mc^2$. The Δm is the mass difference of the nucleus and its constituent particles (protons + neutrons).

Question 8
What are the two types of beta decay? Describe beta decay in general.

Question 9
What is beta minus decay?

Question 10
What is beta plus decay?

Question 11
What is a competing process to beta plus decay?

Answer 8

The two types of beta decay are beta minus decay and beta plus decay. Beta decay is the process by which a radioactive nucleus ejects either a negatively charged electron (beta minus or β^-) or positively charged positron (beta plus or β^+). An electron that is ejected is differentiated from an orbital electron by using the β^- term instead of "e" which refers to an orbital electron. Both forms of beta decay are isobaric as the total atomic number does not change.

Answer 9

In beta minus decay, a neutron is converted into an electron (also known as a β^- particle), a proton, and anti-neutrino. This type of decay is more common with a nucleus that has an n/p ratio >1. The general equation for a beta minus decay is:

$$n \rightarrow p + \beta^- + \bar{\nu}$$

The energy released is the difference in binding energy of the parent and daughter nucleus, minus the mass of the electron. This energy is shared as kinetic energy of the outgoing particles, with on average one third going to the β^- particle, and the remainder to the anti-neutrino ($\bar{\nu}$). The anti-neutrino does not carry any electric charge, and is weakly interacting. There will be an increase in the atomic number of the daughter element by one after a particle undergoes beta minus decay.

Answer 10

Beta plus decay is also known as positron emission and occurs when a radionuclide has a low neutron to proton ratio (n/p) ratio. In beta plus decay, a proton (p) is converted into a positron (also known as a β^+ particle), a neutron (n), and neutrino (ν). The general equation for beta plus decay is:

$$p \rightarrow n + \beta^+ + \nu$$

In beta plus decay, there is a decrease in the atomic number of the daughter element by one. After a beta plus particle is produced, it will eventually interact with an electron causing both particles to be annihilated, producing two photons (gamma rays) that each have energy of 0.511 MeV and travel in opposite directions. Because of this, there is a threshold in the difference between the parent and daughter binding energy of 1.02 MeV for a radionuclide to undergo positron emission.

Answer 11

A competing process to beta plus decay is electron capture. This occurs when the nucleus captures an orbital electron, typically from the K-shell and the proton is converted to a neutron (n), and neutrino (ν). Electron capture does not require a threshold energy of 1.02 MeV to occur and is more prevalent for heavier elements. The general equation for electron capture is:

$$p + e \rightarrow n + \nu$$

Because electron capture leaves an empty hole in the orbital shell, this empty hole can be filled by an outer shell electron, causing a release of a characteristic X-ray or Auger electron. Because electron capture often involves the K shell orbital electron, it is often referred to as K-capture. Similarly to beta plus decay, there will be a decrease in the atomic number of the daughter element by one after a particle undergoes electron capture.

Question 12

What is alpha decay, and describe which radionuclides typically undergo alpha decay?

Question 13

If an isotope $^{220}_{105}A$ decays by α decay and then β^- decay, what is the atomic number and weight of the new element?

Question 1   **1.4 EXPONENTIAL DECAY**

What is the decay constant?

Question 2

What is the time required for either the activity or the number of radioactive atoms to decay to half of the initial value?

Answer 12

Alpha decay is a type of radioactive decay where a nucleus emits an alpha particle. An alpha particle has the same nuclear structure as a helium nucleus. An alpha particle is usually designated by the symbol $^4_2$He. Radionuclides that have a high-Z (usually $Z > 82$) decay most frequently by the emission of an alpha particle. An example of alpha decay is when radium (Ra) undergoes decay to radon (Rn): $^{226}_{88}$Ra $\rightarrow$ $^{222}_{86}$Rn $+ \, ^4_2$He + Energy.

Answer 13

Initial atomic weight is 220, α decay reduces this by 4, β^- decay does not change the number of nucleons. Therefore, the final atomic weight is 216.

The initial atomic number is 105, α decay reduces this by 2, β^- decay increases this by 1, so the final atomic number is 104. The new element is $^{216}_{104}$B.

Answer 1

The decay constant, λ, is a proportionality constant that relates the number of radioactive atom disintegrations per unit time to the number of atoms present. The relationship between the number of remaining atoms (N), to the number of initial atoms (N_0) is related by the exponential equation:

$$N = N_0 e^{-\lambda t}$$

Alternatively this can be written using A as the current activity, and A_0 as the initial activity.

Answer 2

This is the definition of half-life. (Half-Life) $T_{1/2} = \ln(2)/\lambda = (0.693)/\lambda$. After n half-lives, the activity or number of radioactive atoms is reduced to $\frac{1}{2}^n$ of the initial value.

Question 3

What is the average lifetime?

Question 4

What is the specific activity of a radionuclide?

Question 5

The initial activity of an unknown element is 3 Ci. After 12 days, the activity is 2.61 Ci. What is the half-life? What might the element be?

Answer 3

The average or mean lifetime is the average length of time a radioactive atom remains in its sample. Average lifetime (T) equals $1.44 \times$ the half-life ($T_{1/2}$). It is also equivalent to the length of time a sample would take to decay if it continued to decay at its initial decay rate. As such it is useful in calculating dose delivered by permanent implants.

Answer 4

The specific activity of a radionuclide is defined to be its activity per unit mass. The specific activity is independent of the mass of the radionuclide, and has a fixed value independent of the time. The units of specific activity are Ci/g or Bq/kg.

Answer 5

Use the following formula: $A = A_0 \, e^{-0.693t/T_{1/2}}$

$$2.61 = 3 \, e^{-0.693 \times 12/T_{1/2}}$$

$$\ln(2.61/3) = -0.693 \times 12/T_{1/2}$$

$$-0.139 = -8.316/T_{1/2}$$

$$T_{1/2} = 8.316/0.139$$

$$T_{1/2} = 59.7 \text{ days}$$

This is approximately the half-life of I-125. An alternative formula is:

$$T_{1/2} = \frac{-0.693 \, t}{\ln\left(\dfrac{A}{A_0}\right)}$$

Question 6
What is the decay constant of I-125?

Question 7
What is the approximate amount of activity remaining after 1, 2, 3, 4, 5, and 10 half-lives?

Question 8
The initial dose rate of a prostate implant is 7 cGy/hr using I-125 seeds. What is the total dose the prostate will receive?

Question 9
If the initial activity of a new source of Ir-192 for high dose rate (HDR) is about 9.98 Ci, what is the source activity in GBq in three months (90 days) later, given the half-life of Ir-192 is 74 days?

Answer 6
The half-life of I-125 is 59.4 days.

$$\lambda = ln2 / T_{1/2}$$

$$\lambda = \frac{0.693}{59.4}$$

$$= 0.0117 \ d^{-1}$$

Answer 7
After n half-lives, the activity $A = A_0 \ \frac{1}{2}^n$, so

Half-lives	1	2	3	4	5	10
% remaining	50%	25%	12.5%	6.25%	3.125%	~0.1%

These numbers are also relevant when considering the radiation penetrating through n half-value layers of material.

Answer 8
Use the average life of I-125 = 1.44 $T_{1/2}$ = 85.5 days

$$\text{Dose} = \text{initial dose rate} \times \text{average life}$$
$$= 7 \ \text{cGy/hr} \times 85.5 \ \text{days} \times 24 \ \text{hr/day}$$
$$= 14{,}370 \ \text{cGy}.$$

Answer 9
Use the formula:

$$A = A_0 \ e^{-0.693t/T_{1/2}}$$
$$A = 9.98 \ e^{-0.693 \times 90/74}$$
$$A = 9.98 \ e^{-0.843}$$
$$A = 4.30 \ \text{Ci}$$
$$= 4.3 \times 37 \ \text{GBq/Ci}$$
$$= 159 \ \text{GBq}.$$

Question 10
Express the activity formula in terms of number of half-lives and use it to answer the previous question.

Question 11
An high dose rate (HDR) treatment using Ir-192 takes 281 seconds. How long will it take to complete when the patient returns next week for the second fraction?

Question 12
What is the activity of a 30 mCi I-125 prostate implant after one year?

Question 13
A source decays 3% in one day. What is the decrease in activity after 30 days?

Question 14
An Ir-192 high dose rate (HDR) source must have an activity of 10 Ci when it is installed in the afterloader. What activity should it have one week earlier when it is calibrated to ensure this?

Answer 10

The activity formula $A = A_0\, e^{-0.693t/T_{1/2}}$ can be rewritten as:

$$A = A_0 \left(\frac{1}{2}\right)^n$$

where $n = t/T_{1/2}$ is the number of half-lives. This makes the calculation of activity much simpler.

$$\text{Now, } A = 9.98\,(\tfrac{1}{2})^{90/74}$$
$$= 9.98\ 0.5^{1.216}$$
$$= 4.30\ \text{Ci}$$

Answer 11

After seven days, the activity of the source has been reduced by $\tfrac{1}{2}^{7/74}$ or 6.3%. The treatment time must be increased by this amount, $281 \times 1.063 = 299$ sec.

Answer 12

$$A = 30\tfrac{1}{2}^{365/59.4}$$
$$= 0.42\ \text{mCi.}$$

Answer 13

First determine the half-life or decay constant.

$$T_{1/2} = \frac{-0.693\ t}{\ln\left(\dfrac{A}{A_0}\right)}$$

$$T_{1/2} = \frac{-0.693\ 1}{\ln 0.97}$$

$$T_{1/2} = 22.75\ \text{days.}$$
$$A/A_0 = \tfrac{1}{2}^{30/22.75}$$
$$= 0.40$$

So the source activity has decreased by 60% after 30 days.

Answer 14

$$A = A_0 \left(\frac{1}{2}\right)^n$$

$$10\ Ci = A_0 \left(\frac{1}{2}\right)^{7/74}$$

$$A_0 = 10\ /\left(\frac{1}{2}\right)^{7/74}$$

$A_0 = 10.68$ Ci is the activity required at the time of calibration, seven days before.

2

RADIATION GENERATING EQUIPMENT

QINGYANG SHANG AND MATTHEW KOLAR

Question 1

What are the two different mechanisms by which X-rays are produced?

Question 2

Describe how bremsstrahlung and characteristic X-rays are produced.

Question 3

What is the energy spectrum of bremsstrahlung and characteristic X-rays?

Answer 1

X-rays are produced by bremsstrahlung and characteristic X-ray emission. Useful X-ray beams in imaging and therapy are typically all bremsstrahlung, except in mammography where characteristic X-rays are desirable.

Answer 2

Bremsstrahlung X-rays result from the Coulomb interaction between the incident electron and the nuclei of the target material. The incident electron is decelerated, losing kinetic energy in the form of bremsstrahlung photons (radiative loss).

Characteristic X-rays result from Coulomb interactions between the incident electrons and atomic orbital electrons of the target material (collision loss). The orbital electron is ejected from its shell and an electron from a higher level shell fills the vacancy. The energy difference between the two shells may either be emitted from the atom in the form of a characteristic photon (characteristic X-ray) or transferred to another orbital electron that is ejected from the atom as an Auger electron.

Answer 3

Bremsstrahlung X-rays have a spectrum of energies. The maximum X-ray energy is equal to the energy of the incident electron. The energy of the electron corresponds to the peak accelerating voltage. The most probable X-ray energy is about one third of the maximum energy.

Characteristic X-rays have discrete energies, corresponding to the energy level difference between atomic shells involved in the electron transition.

X-ray photons produced by an X-ray tube are the combination of the two. It has a continuous distribution of energies for the bremsstrahlung photons superimposed with characteristic radiation at discrete energies.

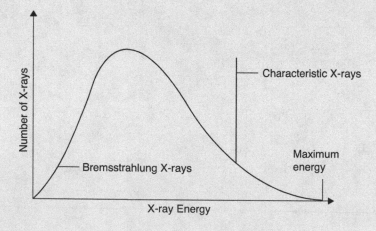

Question 4
What is the classification of therapy X-ray beams?

Question 5
Relative to the incoming electron beam, at what angle are bremsstrahlung X-rays produced?

Question 6
How does fluorescent yield change with Z?

Question 7
How efficient is X-ray production?

Answer 4

X-rays used in radiation oncology are usually classified as:

(a) **Grenz ray therapy**: treatment that uses very low energy (below 20 kV) X-rays. No longer in use.

(b) **Contact therapy**: operates at 40 to 50 kV and facilitates irradiation of accessible lesions at very short source to surface distance (SSD) (2 cm or less). A filter of 0.5- to 1.0-mm-thick aluminum is usually interposed in the beam to absorb the very soft component of the energy spectrum. It is useful for tumors not deeper than 1 to 2 mm.

(c) **Superficial therapy**: treatment with X-rays ranging from 50 to 150 kV. Varying thicknesses of filtration (usually 1–6 mm aluminum) are added to harden the beam to a desired degree. The SSD typically ranges between 15 and 20 cm. Useful for irradiating tumors confined to about 5 mm depth.

(d) **Orthovoltage therapy**: treatment with X-rays ranging from 150 to 500 kV, and filtered with 1 to 4 mm copper. The SSD is typically 50 cm. Useful for tumor less than 2 to 3 cm deep.

(e) **Supervoltage therapy**: X-ray therapy in the range of 500 to 1,000 kV, filtered with 4 to 6 mm copper.

In contrast, diagnostic X-rays are usually in the 10 to 150 kV range.

Answer 5

In the kilovoltage energy range, X-rays are produced uniformly with regards to direction, shielding around the target produces an X-ray beam at 90°. In the megavoltage energy range (1–50 MV) most photons are produced in the direction of electron acceleration (forward direction 0°).

Answer 6

The fluorescent yield ω gives the ratio of fluorescent (characteristic) photons emitted per vacancy in a shell to the number of Auger electrons. It ranges from zero for low-Z atoms through 0.5 for copper ($Z = 29$) to 0.96 for high-Z atoms with K shell vacancies, which are the most prominent sources of characteristic X-rays.

Answer 7

Efficiency of X-ray production is proportional to the atomic number (Z) of target and energy of the electrons. Efficiency is less than 1% for X-ray tubes operating at 100 kVp (99% of input energy is converted into heat). Efficiency improves considerably for megavoltage accelerator beams (30%–95%, depending upon energy).

Question 8
What are the components of a typical X-ray tube?

Question 9
Why is tungsten the chosen material for the cathode and anode of an X-ray tube?

Question 10
What are thin and thick targets, respectively, for an X-ray tube?

Question 11
What is the purpose of the added filtration placed externally to the X-ray tube?

Answer 8

A typical X-ray tube consists of a highly evacuated glass envelope, a cathode (negative electrode, tungsten filament), that produces the electrons, and an anode (positive electrode, tungsten target attached to a thick copper rod).

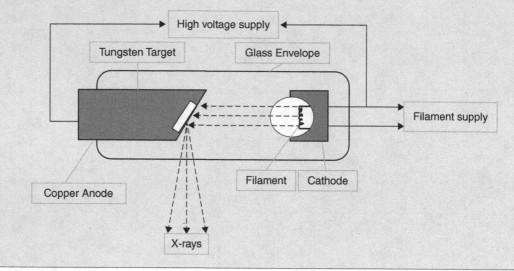

Answer 9

The choice of tungsten for filament (cathode) and target (anode) is based on its high melting point (3,370°C), due to the heat absorbed, and a high atomic number ($Z = 74$) to boost efficiency of X-ray production.

Answer 10

A thin target has a thickness much smaller than R, the range of electrons of a given energy, while the thickness of a thick target is of the order of R.

Answer 11

The purpose of the added filtration is to increase the proportion of high-energy X-rays in the beam by absorbing the lower energy components of the spectrum. Thus, the transmitted beam "hardens" (ie, it achieves higher average energy and therefore greater penetrating power). Another way of improving the penetrating power of the beam is by increasing the voltage across the tube. Since the total intensity of the beam decreases with increasing filtration and increases with voltage, a proper combination of voltage and filtration is required to achieve desired hardening of the beam as well as acceptable intensity.

Question 12

What is half-value layer (HVL)?

Question 13

If a 2 mm thickness of material transmits 25% of a monoenergetic beam of photons, calculate the half-value layer (HVL) and μ of the beam.

Question 14

What is beam hardening?

Question 15

What is heel effect?

Answer 12

HVL is defined as the thickness of material required to reduce the intensity of a beam to one half of its initial value. A related quantity is the linear attenuation coefficient μ, where HVL = $0.693/\mu$.

Answer 13

$$I = I_0 e^{-\mu L}$$

$$0.25 = e^{-\mu \times 0.2 \text{ cm}}$$

$$\mu = -\frac{\ln 0.25}{0.2 \text{ cm}} = 6.93 \text{ cm}^{-1}$$

$$\text{HVL} = \frac{0.693}{\mu} = 0.1 \text{ cm}$$

Answer 14

The lower energy photons of the polyenergetic X-ray beam will be preferentially removed from the beam while passing through matter. The shift of the X-ray spectrum to higher effective energies as the beam transverses matter is called beam hardening. For polyenergetic beams, this causes the second half-value layer (HVL) to be greater than the first HVL.

Answer 15

Since the X-rays are produced at various depths in the target, they suffer varying amounts of attenuation in the target. There is greater attenuation for X-rays coming from greater depths than those from near the surface of the target. Consequently, the intensity of the X-ray beam decreases from the cathode to the anode direction of the beam. This variation across the X-ray beam is called the heel effect. The effect is particularly pronounced in diagnostic tubes because of the low X-ray energy and steep target angles. The problem can be minimized by using a compensating filter to provide differential attenuation across the beam to compensate for the heel effect and improve the uniformity of the beam.

Question 16
What are dual focal spots?

Question 17
The actual anode focal area for a 20° anode angle is 4 mm (length) by 1.2 mm (width). What is the projected focal spot size at the central axis?

Question 18
For an X-ray beam, what is inherent filtration?

Question 19
What is the difference between tube current and filament current?

Question 20
How do tube current (mA) and tube voltage (kVp) affect X-ray intensity?

Answer 16

The size of the target area from which the X-rays are emitted is called the focal spot. The size of the focal spot depends on the size of the tungsten filament of the cathode. In diagnostic radiology, the focal spot should be as small as possible to produce sharp radiographic images. But smaller focal spots generate more heat per unit area of target and thus limit currents and exposure. Diagnostic tubes usually have two separate filaments to provide "dual focus," a small and large filament for small and large images.

Answer 17

An angled target is used to reduce the effective size of the focal spot. The effective focal spot width is equal to the actual focal spot width since it is unaffected by the angle of the anode. The effective focal spot length = actual focal spot length $\times \sin \theta$, where θ is the anode angle.

So for this problem, effective length = 4 mm $\times \sin 20$ = 1.36 mm.

Effective focal spot size = 1.36 mm $\times$ 1.2 mm = 1.632 mm^2

Thus, a large electron beam can be used, to spread the heat on the target, but a small focal spot can be produced for sharp images.

Answer 18

All X-ray beams have some filtration; this is typically from absorption in the target, the wall of the tube and air. This is referred to as inherent filtration.

Answer 19

Filament current is the flow of electrons through the filament. Thermionic emission happens when the filament current is sufficient for electrons to be boiled off and directed toward the anode. Filament current is on the order of amperes (A).

Tube current is the flow of electrons from the cathode to the anode. It is controlled by filament current. A small change in filament current results in an exponential change in tube current. It is on the order of milliampere.

Answer 20

The tube current (mA) is equal to the number of electrons flowing from the cathode to the anode per unit time. Increasing tube current will increase the quantity of electrons available to hit the target, and that results in an increase of X-ray photons produced. Beam on time (seconds) also increases quantity, the combination is mAs.

The tube voltage (kVp) determines the maximum energy in the bremsstrahlung spectrum and affects the quality of the beam. It also affects the efficiency of the X-ray production, which is the number of X-ray photons produced per unit time (quantity). Beam intensity is proportional to kVp^2.
X-ray output is most affected by filament current.

Question 1
How does the flattening filter affect the photon beam?

Question 2
What changes are made to switch from photon mode to electron mode in a linear accelerator (linac)?

Question 3
How does an electron gun work?

Question 4
Why is a bending magnet used in a linear accelerator (linac)?

Question 5
Explain the term isocenter.

Answer 1

The flattening filter is used in photon beams to create a flat dose profile at a depth of 10 cm in water. Without it, the beam profile is very peaked. The flattening filter produces horns at the beam edges at shallower depths. It is typically a conical piece of high-Z material. Due to its introduction to the beam, it increases the effective energy of the beam, by filtering out low energy photons (beam hardening) but it decreases the beam intensity and thus the dose rate.

Answer 2

In electron mode, the target and flattening filter are removed. A scattering foil is added to create a broad, flat beam. An electron applicator is used to collimate the beam by removing the scatter in air. The accelerated beam current is much lower in electron mode, as there is no loss in efficiency as seen in photon mode due to the presence of the target and flattening filter.

Answer 3

An electron gun is a simple electrostatic accelerator containing a heated cathode filament and a perforated grounded anode. A hot cathode emits electrons, which are accelerated toward an anode, passing through an aperture to reach the accelerating waveguide. Along this path, negatively charged focusing electrodes narrow the electrons into a fine beam which then passes through the aperture in the anode. A grid allows for synchronization of electron release into the accelerating waveguide to match its phase.

Answer 4

The bending magnet redirects accelerated electrons toward the isocenter. Using just a 90° bending magnet in the design of a linac allows the accelerator to be oriented parallel to the floor so it can more easily rotate around its isocenter without hitting the ceiling, floor or patient. Using a 270° bending magnet, also allows the energy of electrons to be selected and the electron beam to be focused, thus improving the penumbra of the beam.

Answer 5

Modern linear accelerators (linacs) are constructed so that the axis of gantry rotation, collimator rotation, and table rotation are coincident at one point in space called the isocenter. This allows for a patient to be treated with the isocenter within the target, and have the linac rotate around the patient. Multiple treatment beams can be delivered from various angles without having to the move the patient for each beam.

Question 6

What is the function of the monitor chamber in a linear accelerator (linac)?

Question 7

What is the advantage of a standing wave over a traveling wave accelerating waveguide?

Question 8

Why is sulfur hexafluoride, SF_6 used in a linear accelerator (linac)?

Question 9

What frequency is the accelerating power source for a linear accelerator (linac)?

Question 10

What is a klystron?

Answer 6

It monitors the output of the linac. During linac calibration, charge collected in these ion chambers (represented by monitor units) is correlated to delivered dose. Monitor chambers are then able to turn off the beam once the desired dose has been delivered. Multiple or split chambers are also used to track the flatness and symmetry of the beam.

Answer 7

Standing wave accelerating waveguides are more efficient and shorter than equivalent traveling waveguides. To create a standing wave, the microwaves are reflected at the end, rather than exiting the waveguide. This generates a superposition of the waves in every second cavity, providing double the accelerating power of a traveling wave cavity. The interleaving cavities, where the reflected microwaves cancel are shifted to the side of the electron path as they do not provide any acceleration. Thus, the accelerating power is increased, and the waveguide is shortened.

Answer 8

SF_6 is a dielectric and prevents arcing within the transmission waveguide which guides the microwaves from their source to the accelerating waveguide.

Answer 9

A linac uses microwaves at 3,000 MHz or 3 GHZ. These are called S-band microwaves. Some more compact accelerators, such as CyberKnife, use X-band microwaves around 10 GHz. The size of the waveguide depends on the wavelength of the microwave, so a higher frequency implies a shorter waveguide.

Answer 10

A klystron amplifies low power microwaves into high power microwaves. As electrons are sent though a drift tube, their velocity is modulated by the alternating electric field at the frequency of the entrant low power microwaves, creating "bunches" of electrons. The bunches induce charges on the end cavity, creating higher power microwaves at the same frequency.

Question 11

What is a magnetron?

Question 12

What is the order of components in the head of a linear accelerator (linac)?

Question 13

How would you describe the TomoTherapy system?

Question 14

How would you describe the CyberKnife system?

Question 15

How would you describe the Mobetron?

Answer 11

A magnetron is a microwave generator. It has a circular structure with a cathode at the center and an anode at the outer surface made up of resonant cavities. Electrons are produced at the cathode and are subjected to an electric field between the anode and cathode. A static magnetic field is applied perpendicular to the electric field and motion of the electrons. The electrons move in spirals toward the cavities, creating microwave power, which is then sent to the accelerating waveguide.

Answer 12

The electron beam exits the accelerating waveguide and then is bent by the magnet toward the target. The X-ray beam from the target is shaped by the primary collimator and then the flattening filter, measured by the monitor chamber, and then further shaped by the secondary collimators and multileaf collimators (MLCs).

Answer 13

It is an integrated system with a 6 MV linac mounted in a CT-like ring gantry. An MVCT can be acquired in the treatment position prior to treatment.

Answer 14

CyberKnife features a 6 MV linear accelerator (linac) mounted on an industrial robotic arm. It can position the linac to direct treatment beams from many non-coplanar angles. It also has image guidance (stereoscopic kV and infra-red surface tracking) that continuously monitors the patient's position throughout the treatment process.

Answer 15

The Mobetron is a portable compact electron linear accelerator that is used for intraoperative radiation therapy (IORT). It is self-shielding so it can be used in any operating room. Its treatment energies are 6, 9, or 12 MeV. Because of its short, 50 cm source to surface distance (SSD), the dose rate is quite high (1,000 cGy/min). This leads to short treatment times.

Question 16

The Zeiss intrabeam is a device used for intraoperative radiation therapy (IORT). How are its photons generated?

Question 17

What are some advantages of using a flattening filter free treatment beam?

Question 18

What are the disadvantages of using a flattening filter free treatment beam?

Question 19

How is the wedge angle defined for a physical wedge?

Question 20

How is a wedge transmission factor defined for a physical wedge?

Answer 16

The electron gun injects electrons into the accelerator with a maximum voltage of 50 kV. The electrons are directed to a gold target which is placed at the center of a spherical acrylic applicator. X-rays of approximately 20 keV are emitted isotropically.

Answer 17

The dose rate can be three to five times higher, which results in faster treatments. The absence of a flattening filter significantly reduces the amount of scattered radiation. This can reduce the total body dose to the patient and also make it easier to model the beam in a treatment planning system.

Answer 18

The beam profile is forward peaked. The beam is only meant to treat small targets. Very large targets would require more monitor units to treat the tumor volume that is far away from the central axis. The beam is also slightly less penetrating than a flattened beam which is hardened by the presence of the flattening filter.

Answer 19

Wedge angle is usually defined as the angle of the 50% isodose curve with respect to the central axis at a reference depth of 10 cm.

Answer 20

The wedge transmission factor is defined as the ratio of the dose with the wedge present to the dose without the wedge present at a depth of 10 cm.

Question 21

What are the different methods for obtaining a wedged isodose distribution?

Question 22

How does the inverse square law relate to absorbed dose from a linear accelerator (linac)?

Question 23

A photon field is calculated for 100 cm source to surface distance (SSD). If the patient is setup at 110 cm SSD, what error would you estimate for the delivered dose?

Question 24

A post-spine treatment calculation is changed from 10 cm depth and 100 cm source to surface distance (SSD) to 10 cm depth source to axis distance (SAD). How will the calculation change? Will the monitor units increase or decrease?

Question 25

What is a double-focused multileaf collimator (MLC)?

Answer 21

The Physical Wedge is a tray-mounted block of steel, placed in the accessory slot of a linear accelerator (linac). The steel is shaped like a wedge, with one end thicker than the other. The thicker end, known as the heel, modulates the beam more than the other end, the toe. Physical wedges are available in fixed, standard angles, usually 15°, 30°, 45°, and 60°.

The Universal Wedge is similar to a 60° physical wedge, but it is integrated into the head of the linac. The wedge moves in and out of the treatment beam, depending upon the desired wedge isodose angle. A 60° wedge isodose angle would require that the wedge be in the beam for the duration of the treatment field. For a lower wedge isodose angle, the wedge would move out of the treatment field for a fraction of the treatment.

The Dynamic Wedge creates a wedged isodose angle by moving the collimator jaw across the field. The wedge isodose angle can be changed by modulating the dose rate and/or changing the speed of the jaw.

The multileaf collimator (MLC) can be used with segmented fields to create any dose distribution.

Answer 22

The absorbed dose factor is inversely proportional to the square of the distance from the target. This is due to the divergence of the beam. Imagine a sphere around the target with radius r. The surface of the sphere is $4\pi r^2$, with all the radiation from the target passing through it. Now imagine a sphere twice as far away from the target, the same amount of radiation will pass through its surface, but the surface area is four times the size, effectively reducing the intensity at any one point by four.

Answer 23

Inverse Square Law: $100^2/110^2 = 0.83$
The patient would be underdosed by 17%

Answer 24

The SSD factor is replaced with a SAD factor and the percentage depth dose (PDD) is replaced with tissue maximum ratio (TMR). The monitor units will decrease as the patient is 10 cm closer to the source.

Answer 25

In a double-focused MLC, the divergence of the MLC matches that of the treatment beam in the x and y directions. In one direction, the leaves move in an arcing direction to match the leaf ends with the beam divergence. In the other direction, the divergence is matched by varying the cross-sectional width of the leaves. The leaves are made thinner at the end closer to the target. Both of these result in a sharper penumbra.

Question 1   **2.3 PARTICLE AND SOURCE-BASED RADIATION**
How long is the half-life of cobalt-60 (Co-60)?

Question 2
How would you describe the decay scheme for cobalt-60 (Co-60)?

Question 3
What is the difference between electrostatic and cyclic accelerators?

Question 4
What are some examples of electrostatic accelerators and cyclic accelerators used in medicine?

Answer 1

The half-life $T_{1/2}$ (the time required for the activity of the source to be halved) of Co-60 is 5.27 years. For practical purposes it is considered harmless and inactive after 10 half-lives. Thus, Co-60 would need to be stored safely for approximately 53 years.

Answer 2

A cobalt-60 nucleus is produced in a nuclear reactor by bombarding stable Co-59 atoms with neutrons. To decay to a stable state, the Co-60 nucleus first emits a β^- particle (β^- decay) and then, two gamma emissions with energies of 1.17 and 1.33 MeV are observed. The average energy of the gammas is 1.25 MeV.

Creation: $^{59}_{27}\text{Co} + ^{1}_{0}n \rightarrow ^{60}_{27}\text{Co} + \gamma$

Decay: $^{60}_{27}\text{Co} \xrightarrow{T_{1/2}} ^{60}_{28}\text{Ni} + ^{0}_{-1}\beta + \gamma_1 + \gamma_2$

Answer 3

In electrostatic accelerators, the particles are accelerated by a constant electrostatic field over a voltage difference. The kinetic energy that the particle can gain is limited by the maximum voltage difference of the electrostatic field.

In cyclic accelerators, the electric fields are variable and particles repeatedly pass through them. This requires increasingly strong magnetic fields or radii of curvature to keep the particles returning to the cavity.

Answer 4

Examples of electrostatic accelerators used in medicine are superficial and orthovoltage X-ray tubes and neutron generators. Examples of cyclic accelerators are microtrons, betatrons, cyclotrons, and synchrotrons.

Question 5

What are examples of megavoltage radiation therapy machines?

Question 6

What is a betatron, a microtron, and a cyclotron?

Question 7

What is the advantage of proton and heavy charged particle radiation compared to photon and electron beams?

Question 8

How is the range for other charged particles calculated given the range of protons with the same initial velocity?

Answer 5

Examples of clinical megavoltage machines are accelerators such as Van de Graaff generator, linear accelerator (linac), betatron, cyclotron and microtron, and teletherapy gamma ray units such as cobalt-60.

Answer 6

Cyclotron: A circular accelerator where charged particles generated at a central source are accelerated spirally outward in a plane perpendicular to a fixed magnetic field by an alternating electrical field. A cyclotron is capable of generating particle energies of between 1 and 30 MeV.

Betatron: Developed in 1940 for the circular induction acceleration of electrons and light particles. The magnetic field guide is increased over time to keep the particles in a constant-diameter circle. Mean energy is 45 MeV (maximum energy ~300 MeV). After the advent of linear accelerators (linacs) they have not been used due to their large dimensions, high costs, and low dose rates.

Microtron: Entered clinics in 1972 as a combination of a linear accelerator, followed by magnets to bend the electrons around to re-enter the accelerator. It can produce electrons energies of up to 50 MeV. One microtron generator is used to provide electrons for more than one treatment room.

	Magnetic Field	**Electric Field**
Cyclotron	Constant	Alternating
Betatron	Variable	Vortex
Microtron	Fixed	Variable

Answer 7

The major advantage of high-energy protons and other heavy charged particles is their characteristic dose distribution as a function of depth. As the beam traverses the tissues, the dose deposited is approximately constant with depth until near the end of the range where the dose peaks followed by a rapid falloff to zero. The region of high dose at the end of the particle range is called the Bragg peak.

Answer 8

The approximate range for other particles with the same initial velocity can be calculated by the following relationship:

$$R_1 / R_2 = \left(M_1 / M_2\right) \times \left(Z_2 / Z_1\right)^2$$

where R_1 and R_2 are particle ranges, M_1 and M_2 are the masses, and Z_1 and Z_2 are the charges of the two particles being compared. Thus, from the range energy data for protons one can calculate the range of other particles such as alphas and carbon ions.

Question 9
How are neutron beams produced?

Question 10
How would you describe the decay scheme for radium?

Question 11
How would you describe the depth dose curve of a clinical electron beam?

Answer 9

High-energy neutron beams for radiation therapy are produced by bombarding a target with charged particles from a cyclotron or linear accelerator or in a deuterium–tritium (D–T) generator. As neutrons have no electric charge, they cannot be steered or focused. The produced neutrons travel mainly in the direction of the incoming particles. The bombarding particles are either deuterons (D) or protons hitting a target usually made of beryllium, except in the D–T generator in which tritium (T) is used as the target.

Answer 10

Radium decays to radon through alpha emission. An alpha particle is ejected with energy of 4.78 MeV or 4.6 MeV. The 4.6 MeV alpha particle is accompanied by a 0.18 MeV gamma ray.

$$^{226}_{88}\text{Ra} \rightarrow \, ^{222}_{86}\text{Rn} + \, ^{4}_{2}\text{He}$$

Answer 11

Surface dose is high for electron beams followed by a gradual curve up until the depth of maximum dose (d_{max}). The depth of maximum dose increases with increasing energy. Beyond d_{max}, the depth dose decreases very rapidly. R50 is defined as the depth at which the dose deposited is half the maximum dose. Practical range or Rp, is defined as the point of intersection at which the depth dose curve is extrapolated down to the bremsstrahlung tail.

3

IONIZING RADIATION

ZHILEI LIU SHEN AND TOUFIK DJEMIL

Question 1

What are the five major types of photon interactions with matter?

Question 2

What is Rayleigh scattering?

Question 3

What is the photoelectric effect?

Question 4

What is Compton scattering?

Answer 1

The five major types of photon interactions with matter in order of energy threshold are (1) Rayleigh scattering, also known as coherent scattering, classical scattering, or elastic scattering; (2) photoelectric effect, also known as photoelectric absorption; (3) Compton scattering, also known as incoherent scattering, or Compton effect; (4) pair production; and (5) photodisintegration or photonuclear.

Answer 2

In Rayleigh scattering, the incident photon interacts with the atom as a whole, scattering off in a different direction without losing energy.

Answer 3

In the photoelectric effect, the entire energy of the incident photon is transferred to an orbital electron, which is then ejected from the atom. The energy of the ejected electron (photoelectron) is the energy of the incident photon minus the binding energy. Characteristic X-ray or Auger electron emission will subsequently occur, filling the vacancy of the photoelectron.

Answer 4

Compton scattering is a collision between a photon and a loosely bound outer shell orbital electron of an atom, resulting in a scattered photon of lower energy and an electron. This is the dominant interaction of therapeutic X-ray beams with tissue. Because the incident photon energy greatly exceeds the binding energy of the outer shell electron, the Compton interaction looks like a collision between the photon and a free electron (termed nearly free).

Question 5

What is pair production?

Question 6

What is photodisintegration?

Question 7

With one incoming photon, what are the outgoing particles produced during Rayleigh scattering, photoelectric effect, Compton scattering, and pair production, respectively?

Question 8

Does ionization occur in Rayleigh scattering?

Answer 5

In pair production, the photon interacts strongly with the electromagnetic field of an atomic nucleus and gives up all of its energy to create an electron and a positron.

Answer 6

In photodisintegration, an incident photon with high energy (>7 to 10 MeV) collides with the nucleus of an atom and all of the photon's energy gets absorbed. The nucleus then emits a neutron. This effect causes extra shielding requirements for high-energy beams.

Answer 7

With one incoming photon, the outgoing particles produced by the four photon interactions are listed as follows:

Rayleigh scattering: one photon
Photoelectric effect: one electron
Compton scattering: one electron and one photon
Pair production: one electron and one positron

Answer 8

Ionization does not occur in Rayleigh scattering because electrons are not ejected.

Question 9

What is the dependence of the photoelectric effect on atomic number (Z) and energy (E)?

Question 10

What is the dependence of Compton scattering on atomic number (Z), energy (E), and electron density (N_e)?

Question 11

What is the dependence of pair production on atomic number (Z) and energy (E)?

Question 12

Is Compton scattering most likely to occur with inner or outer shell electrons?

Answer 9

The photoelectric effect is proportional to Z^3/E^3, where Z is the atomic number of the target atom, and E is the energy of the incident photon.

Answer 10

The probability of Compton scattering is independent of Z and decreases with E. Compton scattering depends on the electron density N_e of the material.

Answer 11

The probability of pair production changes with Z^2 and $\log(E)$.

Answer 12

Compton scattering is most likely to occur with outer shell electrons.

Question 13

What is the minimum energy of an incident photon for the pair-production process?

Question 14

Which interaction is the main cause for the absorption in water of photons with energy 10 to 100 keV?

Question 15

Which interaction is the main cause for the absorption in water of photons with energy 100 keV to 10 MeV?

Question 16

When is the photoelectric effect most probable with respect to the energy of the photon and the electron binding energy?

Answer 13

The minimum energy of an incident photon for the pair-production process is 1.02 MeV. This energy corresponds to the mass of the electron and positron produced (0.511 MeV each). Additional energy above the 1.02 MeV threshold is carried away as kinetic energy by the pair.

Answer 14

Photoelectric effect is the main cause for the absorption in water of photons with energy 10 to 100 keV. This is the range of diagnostic X-rays. The dependence of the absorption on atomic number Z^3 provides the excellent contrast of diagnostic X-ray images.

Answer 15

Compton scattering is the main cause for the absorption in water of photons with energy of 100 keV–10 MeV. This is the range of therapeutic X-rays.

Answer 16

The photoelectric effect is most probable when the energy of the photon is slightly higher than the electron binding energy. In the absorption spectrum, the shell binding energies appear as sharp peaks known as "absorption edges," labeled by the corresponding shell, for example, K-edge, for absorption from the inner most shell.

Question 17

What is KERMA?

Question 18

At what energy are the probabilities of Compton scattering and photoelectric effect about the same for soft tissue?

Question 19

In Compton scattering, a 6 MeV incident photon scatters to 60°, what is the energy of the ejected Compton electron?

Question 20

In Compton scattering, as the incident photon energy increases, are the photons and electrons scattered more toward the forward or backward direction?

Answer 17
KERMA is the Kinetic Energy Released per unit MAss. This represents the energy transferred to the medium by the photon.

Answer 18
The probabilities of Compton scattering and photoelectric effect are about the same at ~30 keV for soft tissue.

Answer 19
In Compton scattering, the energy of the scattered photon can be calculated as

$$E_{sc} = \frac{E_0}{1 + \dfrac{E_0}{511 \text{ keV}}(1 - \cos\theta)}$$

where E_{sc} is the energy of the scattered photon, E_0 is the energy of the incident photon, and θ is the angle of the scattered photon with respect to the incident trajectory. Therefore, the energy of the scattered photon is ~873 keV.

The kinetic energy of the ejected Compton electron (E_e) can be calculated as

$$E_e = E_0 - E_{sc}.$$

Therefore, the energy of the ejected Compton electron is ~5.13 MeV.

Answer 20
In Compton scattering, as the incident photon energy increases, both photons and electrons are scattered more toward the forward direction. Additionally, the proportion of energy carried by the scattered electron increases with incident photon energy.

Question 21

In Compton scattering, what are the maximal energies of a photon scattered through 90° and 180°?

Question 22

A 200 keV incident photon undergoes the photoelectric effect with an iodine atom and a K-shell electron is ejected. What is the kinetic energy of the ejected photoelectron given that the K-shell binding energy is 34 keV?

Question 23

Given the binding energies of the K-, L-, M-, N-shell electrons of an iodine atom are 34, 5, 0.6, and ~0 keV, respectively, what are the energies of the characteristic X-rays following the ejection of a K-shell electron?

Answer 21

In Compton scattering, the maximal energy of the scattered photon is 511 keV at 90° and 255 keV at 180° (ie, backscatter). These are energies of interest for secondary shielding.

Answer 22

In the photoelectric effect, the kinetic energy of the ejected photoelectron (E_e) can be calculated as

$$E_e = E_0 - E_b$$

where E_0 is the energy of the incident photon (200 keV in this case), E_b is the binding energy of the orbital electron (34 keV). Therefore, the kinetic energy of the ejected photoelectron is 200 − 34 = 166 keV.

Answer 23

The vacancy created in the K-shell causes the transition of an electron from a higher shell to the K-shell. This may create in an intermediate shell (eg, L or M) that can be filled from an even higher shell electron. This electron cascade continues as outer shell electrons jump to inner shells. The difference in their binding energies is released as either characteristic X-rays or Auger electrons. In this case, the energies of the characteristic X-rays are ~34 keV (N–K), 33.4 keV (M–K), 29 keV (L–K), ~5 keV (N–L), 4.4 keV (M–L), and ~0.6 keV (N–M).

Question 1

What are some examples of charged and uncharged particles?

Question 2

What are the three types of interactions that a charged particle can have with the matter?

Question 3

What is the difference between excitation and ionization?

Question 4

What are some examples of ionizing and nonionizing radiations?

Answer 1

Alpha particles (α^{2+} or He^{2+}), protons (p^+), beta particles (β^-), positrons (β^+), and electrons (e^-) are some examples of charged particles. Photons (ie, X-ray and gamma-ray), neutrons, and neutrinos are some examples of uncharged particles.

Answer 2

There are excitation, ionization, and bremsstrahlung. Excitation and ionization are interactions of the charged particle with the orbital electrons. Bremsstrahlung is an interaction of the charged particle with the nucleus.

Answer 3

The main difference between excitation and ionization is whether an orbital electron is ejected from the atom. In excitation, the transferred energy does not exceed the binding energy of the electron, so the electron is raised to a higher energy level without actual ejection. In ionization, the transferred energy exceeds the binding energy of the electron, so the electron is ejected from the atom.

Answer 4

X-rays, gamma-rays, electrons, protons, alpha particles, and neutrons are some examples of ionizing radiation. Microwaves, radio waves, and optical photons are some examples of nonionizing radiation.

Question 5
What are the differences between directly and indirectly ionizing radiation?

Question 6
What are delta rays?

Question 7
What is specific ionization (SI)?

Question 8
What is the dependence of specific ionization (SI) on the charge (Q) and velocity (v) of the incident charged particle?

Answer 5

Directly ionizing radiation comes from charged particles (eg, protons, electrons, and alpha particles) and indirectly ionizing radiation from uncharged particles (eg, photons and neutrons).

Answer 6

Delta rays are secondary electrons with sufficient energy to travel a significant distance away from the primary radiation beam and produce further ionization (ie, secondary ionization).

Answer 7

The average number of primary and secondary ion pairs produced per unit length of the charged particle's path is called the SI. SI is often expressed in units of ion pairs per mm (IP/mm).

Answer 8

SI increases with Q^2 and decreases with v^2. Thus, SI $\propto Q^2/v^2$.

Question 9

What is the Bragg peak?

Question 10

What is the difference between the path length and range of a particle?

Question 11

What is the linear energy transfer (LET)?

Question 12

What is the dependence of linear energy transfer (LET) on the charge (Q) and kinetic energy (E_k) of the incident charged particle?

Answer 9

As a charged particle travels through matter, it loses velocity causing its specific ionization (SI) to increase to a maximum (called the Bragg peak) when it stops. The SI drops off rapidly after the proton has deposited its energy.

Answer 10

The path length of a particle is the distance that the particle travels, while the range of a particle is the depth of penetration of the particle in matter. The path length of an individual electron almost always exceeds its range, while the path length of a heavy charged particle (eg, alpha particles) is essentially equal to its range.

Answer 11

The LET is the average amount of energy deposited locally in matter per unit path length. LET is often expressed in units of keV per μm (keV/μm).

Answer 12

The LET of a charged particle increases with Q^2 and decreases with E_k. Thus, LET $\propto Q^2/E_k$.

Question 13

What are some examples of high linear energy transfer (LET) and low LET radiation?

Question 14

What is a bremsstrahlung X-ray?

Question 15

What is the dependence of bremsstrahlung on the atomic number (Z) of the absorber and the mass (m) of the incident particle?

Question 16

What is positron annihilation?

Answer 13

Alpha particles, protons, and neutrons are examples of high LET radiation. Electrons, X-rays, and gamma-rays are examples of low LET.

Answer 14

As an electron interacts with an atomic nucleus, it is deflected and decelerated by the positively charged nucleus, with a loss of kinetic energy as emission of bremsstrahlung X-rays. Bremsstrahlung is a German word meaning "braking radiation."

Answer 15

Total bremsstrahlung emission per atom increases with Z^2 and decreases with m^2.
Thus, bremsstrahlung $\propto Z^2/m^2$.

Answer 16

A positron interacts with an electron at the end of its range, resulting in the annihilation of the electron–positron pair and the conversion of their rest mass to energy in the form of two oppositely directed 0.511 MeV photons.

Question 17

What is the stopping power of a charged particle?

Question 18

What is the mass stopping power of a charged particle?

Question 19

What are the two types of stopping power, according to how the energy is lost by the charged particle?

Question 20

What are the relative speeds of alpha particles (α^{2+}), protons (p^+), and electrons (e^-) with the same energy from the slowest to the fastest?

Answer 17

The stopping power of a charged particle is the energy loss per unit of path length in a medium, usually given in units of MeV/m or joule (J/m).

Answer 18

The mass stopping power of a charged particle is the stopping power divided by the density of the medium, usually given in units of MeV m^2/kg or J m^2/kg.

Answer 19

According to the fate of the energy lost by the charged particle, the stopping power may be divided into "collisional stopping power" from excitation and ionization, and "radiative stopping power" from bremsstrahlung.

Answer 20

$\alpha^{2+} < p^+ < e^-$. Kinetic energy depends on mass and speed squared. For the same energy, the lightest particle will be fastest, so the rank follows the mass of the particles.

Question 21

What are the relative ranges of alpha particles (α^{2+}), protons (p^+), and electrons (e^-) with the same energy from the longest to the shortest?

Question 22

Which key feature allows proton and heavier charged particle beams to concentrate dose inside the tumor target while minimizing dose to the surrounding normal tissues?

Question 23

What are two main types of neutron interactions with matter?

Question 24

Do neutrons directly cause excitation and ionization?

Answer 21

$e^- > p^+ > \alpha^{2+}$. Range is proportional to mass and inversely proportional to charge squared.

Answer 22

As charged particles slow down, they release more energy to the medium, this property causes the Bragg peak, a large deposit of energy at the end of the particle's range.

Answer 23

The two main types of neutron interactions with matter are scattering and absorption. Neutrons may interact with nuclei via scattering in "billiard ball"-like collisions, producing recoil nuclei that deposit their energy via excitation and ionization. Neutrons may also be absorbed by nuclei and cause a variety of emissions, such as gamma-rays, charged particles, neutrons, or fission fragments.

Answer 24

No, neutrons do not directly cause excitation and ionization. Neutrons are uncharged particles, so they do not interact with electrons via excitation and ionization.

Question 25

How many ion pairs can a 1 MeV secondary electron produce given that the energy required to produce an ion pair in soft tissue is ~22 eV?

Question 26

What is the Cerenkov effect?

Question 27

How frequently does the Cerenkov effect occur?

Answer 25

The number of ion pairs produced by a 1 MeV secondary electron is $(1 \times 10^6 \text{ eV})/22 \text{ eV} \approx 45454$.

Answer 26

The Cerenkov effect occurs when a charged particle travels in a medium at a speed greater than the speed of light in that medium (no massive particle can travel faster than light in a vacuum). Under this condition, the charged particle creates an electromagnetic "shock wave," similar to the acoustic shock wave when an airplane travels faster than the sound speed. The electromagnetic shock wave appears as a burst of visible radiation, referred to as Cerenkov radiation. Potentially this could be used to measure the position and intensity of deposited dose.

Answer 27

The probability of the Cerenkov effect occurring is very small (much less than 1%), but some patients receiving electron treatment near their eyes may describe seeing bluish rings during treatment.

4

ABSORBED DOSE

MARTIN ANDREWS AND NAICHANG YU

Question 1

What is the definition of exposure?

Question 2

Why is the concept of exposure not suitable for dosimetry of megavoltage beams?

Question 3

What is the definition of the roentgen (R)? Express this quantity in SI units.

Question 4

What is the f factor for absorbed dose?

Question 5

How is the f factor used to calculate absorbed dose?

Answer 1
Exposure is defined as the quotient $\frac{dQ}{dm}$, where dQ is the total charge of ions of one sign that are produced in air when all charged particles produced by photons are completely stopped, and dm is the mass of air within which the charged particles are liberated.

Answer 2
The definition of exposure requires that charged particles are completely stopped in air. For megavoltage beams, the range of charged particles in air is too large for measurement of exposure to be practical.

Answer 3
The R is the unit of exposure. The original unit was defined as the amount of radiation that liberates 1 esu (electrostatic unit) of charge per cubic centimeter of air. To express the roentgen in SI units, we use the conversion factor for esu to C (Coulombs) and the density of air (approximately 1.293 kg/m³). Since 1 esu $\approx 3.34 \times 10^{-10}$ C, we have

$$1R = 1\ \frac{esu}{cm^3} \rightarrow \frac{1\ esu \times 3.34 \times 10^{-10}\ \frac{C}{esu}}{1\ cm^3 \times 1.293\ \frac{kg}{m^3} \times \frac{m^3}{10^6 cm^3}} = 2.58 \times 10^{-4}\ \frac{C}{kg}$$

Answer 4
The f factor is used to convert exposure, which is only defined in air, to dose in a medium. It is termed the roentgen to rad factor. For air, f is 0.876.

Answer 5
Assuming that charged particle equilibrium (CPE) exists at the point of interest; dose in the medium can be calculated using the formula:

$$D_m(cGy) = f \times X \times \frac{\Psi_m}{\Psi_{air}}$$

where X is the exposure (R) and $\frac{\Psi_m}{\Psi_{air}}$ is the energy fluence ratio in the medium m to that of air. The f factor of water ranges from 0.0.88 to 0.97 depending on the energy of the X-rays.

Question 6
Explain why the R-to-cGy conversion factor, f, is material and energy dependent.

Question 7
What is absorbed dose? What is its unit?

Question 8
Does absorbed dose uniquely specify the biological effect on tissues?

Question 9
What theory relates the charge collected in an ionization chamber to the dose delivered to the medium around the chamber?

Question 10
According to the Bragg–Gray cavity theory, how is the dose to the medium surrounding the chamber related to the dose to the air inside the chamber?

Answer 6

The f factor is defined as:

$$f = 0.876 \frac{(\bar{\mu}_{en} / \rho)_m}{(\bar{\mu}_{en} / \rho)_{air}}$$

The numerator of this expression contains the average mass energy absorption coefficient for the material of interest. Different materials have different interaction cross sections and hence f is inherently medium dependent. The mass energy absorption coefficient is also energy dependent since different interaction processes dominate in different energy domains. Recall from Question 4 that 0.876 is the f factor for air.

Answer 7

Absorbed dose is the energy absorbed per unit mass. This is a physically measurable quantity. Its standard unit is the gray (Gy), which is 1 joule (J) of energy absorbed by 1 kg of mass.

Answer 8

The biological effect of radiation on tissue is not uniquely determined by the absorbed dose. It may depend on other qualities of the radiation such as the type of radiation and the rate the radiation is delivered.

Answer 9

Bragg–Gray cavity theory relates the number of ions collected in an ion chamber to the dose delivered in a medium in which the chamber is placed.

Answer 10

The mean ratio of mass stopping powers of the medium and the gas inside the chamber is the same as the ratio of dose in the medium to dose in the gas.

Question 11

What two assumptions are part of the Bragg–Gray cavity theory?

Question 12

How does Spencer–Attix cavity theory differ from Bragg–Gray cavity theory?

Question 13

What is charged particle equilibrium (CPE)?

Question 14

What equation is used for calibration of linear accelerators in the TG-51 protocol? Briefly describe each of the terms and its units.

Answer 11

First, the presence of the cavity medium does not affect the charged particle field because its thickness is small compared to the range of charged particles impinging on it. Second, all the dose in the cavity medium is deposited by the charged particles traversing it.

Answer 12

Spencer–Attix cavity theory instead uses the restricted mass stopping power with a cutoff value of Δ (typically 10–20 keV) to take into account the effect of delta rays. Spencer–Attix is therefore more accurate.

Answer 13

CPE is the concept that given a volume V, every charged particle of one sign and energy exiting V is, on average, replaced by an identical charged particle of the same energy entering V.

Answer 14

$$D_W^Q = N_{D,w}^{60_{Co}} M k_Q$$

where D_W^Q is the absorbed dose to water measured at the reference point in a beam of quality Q. Its unit is the Gy.

$N_{D,w}^{60_{Co}}$ is the calibration coefficient for converting measured charge to dose. It has units of Gy/C.

M is the fully corrected electrometer reading, in units of C.

k_Q is a quality conversion factor which corrects the calibration coefficient for differences in beam quality between the beam which is being calibrated and a ^{60}Co beam. It is unitless.

Question 15
How do you compute the temperature and pressure correction factor described in TG-51?

Question 16
Why is the temperature and pressure correction necessary?

Question 17
What is the result of performing the TG-51 protocol?

Question 18
What is the typical calibration geometry?

Question 19
Why does changing the polarity of the voltage applied to an ion chamber affect its response?

Answer 15

TG-51 defines the temperature and pressure correction factor as:

$$P_{T,P} = \frac{760}{P} \times \frac{273.2 + T}{295.2}$$

where P is the atmospheric pressure in units of mmHg. For P given in units of kPa, the conversion 1 kPa = 7.5 mmHg must be used. The temperature T in °C is converted to kelvin (K) by adding 273.2, and 295.2 is the temperature in K under reference conditions.

Answer 16

For unsealed ion chambers, response can change because the mass of air within the chamber varies with pressure and temperature. $P_{T,P}$ corrects for deviations of temperature and pressure from reference conditions (295.2 K and 760 mmHg) under which the chamber was calibrated.

Answer 17

The TG-51 protocol provides a means for calibrating the output of a linear accelerator. The result is the calibration of dose to monitor units (MUs) at one specific point in a water phantom, at one distance, for one field size.

Answer 18

Typically, the calibration geometry is a reference field size of 10 cm × 10 cm, 100 cm distance from the source to the surface of water, and at the nominal maximum depth of the energy calibrated. Determination of dose at other points can then be calculated based on measured output factors, for example, tissue-maximum ratio (TMR), collimator scatter factor (Sc), phantom scatter factor (Sp), off-axis ratio (OAR), percent depth dose (PDD), and so on.

Answer 19

The charge measured by the electrometer depends on the polarity applied to the ion chamber. Photons interact not only with the gas in the ion chamber but also with the central electrode, ejecting electrons which may increase or decrease depending on the polarity applied to the ion chamber. Additional current outside the collection cavity, known as extra-cameral current, may also occur due to poorly screened circuitry or interactions that take place in the ion chamber cable.

Question 20

Why do ion chambers need to be corrected for ion recombination?

Question 21

In the TG-51 protocol, how is the electrometer correction factor determined?

Question 22

Suppose 1 g of water, 1 g of air, and 1 g of polystyrene each absorbs 1 J of energy. In which of these media is the absorbed dose the highest?

Question 23

Which treatment would you expect to result in more dose to the skin, 10 MV photons or 10 MeV electrons?

Question 24

Water equivalent phantoms are frequently used in radiation therapy. What is the necessary condition for a phantom to be water equivalent?

Answer 20

An ion chamber's high voltage is used to separate and collect ions that form in the presence of ionizing radiation. The collection process is not 100% efficient and some ions will recombine before reaching the electrodes, thereby causing loss of signal.

Answer 21

The electrometer correction factor, P_{elec}, is necessary when the ion chamber and electrometer are not calibrated as a unit. This factor is provided by an Accredited Dosimetry Calibration Laboratory (ADCL), and must be rechecked by the ADCL every two years.

Answer 22

Absorbed dose is defined as the energy absorbed per unit mass. Since each medium absorbs the same amount of energy and also contains the same mass, they all receive the same dose.

Answer 23

Skin dose from electron beams is higher than that from photon beams. High-energy photon beams (>1 MV) are indirectly ionizing and therefore deposit their dose downstream, in a few cm depth. Electron beams, however, are directly ionizing. The electrons in an electron beam can deposit significant dose directly at the patient's surface.

Answer 24

Photon absorption is based on electron density and the atomic number. A water-equivalent phantom must have the same electron density (number of electrons per cm³ 3.34×10^{23} for water) and effective atomic number, $Z_{eff} = 7.42$.

Question 25
What is the definition of KERMA?

Question 26
What are the components of kinetic energy released per unit mass (KERMA)?

Question 1   **4.2 DOSIMETERS**
What characteristics should an ideal dosimeter have?

Question 2
What types of dosimeters are considered absolute dosimeters (ie, they do not need to be calibrated before absolute dose can be measured)?

Question 3
How do free-air ionization chambers work?

Answer 25

KERMA is an acronym which stands for "kinetic energy released per unit mass." It is defined as the ratio

$$\frac{dE_{tr}}{dm}$$

where dE_{tr} is the total initial kinetic energy of all charged particles set in motion by photons in a mass dm of material. KERMA can also be calculated as:

$$\psi\left(\frac{\overline{\mu_{tr}}}{\rho}\right)$$

Where $\dfrac{\overline{\mu_{tr}}}{\rho}$ is the mean mass energy transfer coefficient and Ψ is the photon energy fluence. KERMA is expressed in units of J/kg.

Answer 26

KERMA can be broken down into collision (depositing dose) and radiative (bremsstrahlung) components.

Answer 1

An ideal dosimeter should be able to measure the radiation dose accurately, with the same sensitivity regardless of the type of radiation, energy of the radiation, dose rate, or exposure history of the dosimeter.

Answer 2

There are three common types of absolute dosimeters: free-air ionization chambers, Fricke ferrous sulfate dosimeters, and calorimeters.

Answer 3

Free-air ionization chambers are large ionization chambers designed to measure exposure. Their large size and energy limitations mostly confine their use to national standards laboratories.

Question 4

Calculate the temperature change if 1 g of water absorbs a dose of 1 Gy. How many Gy are required to raise the temperature of 1 g of water at 25°C to its boiling point at 100°C? The specific heat capacity of water is 4.18 J g^{-1} °C^{-1}.

Question 5

How do ion chambers work?

Question 6

What bias voltage is applied to an ion chamber?

Answer 4

Calorimeters work on the principle that most of the energy absorbed in a medium will wind up as heat. The resulting rise in temperature needs to be accurately measured to calculate the absorbed dose. This is the most direct measurement of dose.

Temperature change can be computed as: $Q = m \times c \times \Delta T$, where Q is the amount of heat energy, c is the specific heat capacity, and ΔT is the change in temperature. Since 1 Gy = 1 J/kg of absorbed energy, we have for water:

$$Q = 1 \frac{J}{kg} \times \frac{1 \text{ kg}}{1000 \text{ g}} \times 1\text{ g} = 0.001 \text{ J}$$

The change in temperature can be computed from:

$$\Delta T = \frac{Q}{m \times c} = \frac{0.001 \text{ J}}{4.18 \text{ J g}^{-1}{}^{\circ}\text{C}^{-1} \times 1 \text{ g}} = 2.39 \times 10^{-4}{}^{\circ}\text{C}$$

This illustrates that 1 Gy of radiation therapy produces a very small change in temperature. Calorimetry is therefore a very difficult method of measuring dose for the calibration of treatment machinery.

Answer 5

The figure is a cross section of an ion chamber. Usually the chamber consists of two conducting poles and a space between the poles filled with air. Radiation ionizes the air molecules and makes electron and positive-ion pairs. These charged particles are driven by the bias voltage to the two poles and are collected by the electrometer. The number of ion pairs produced and therefore the charge collected on the poles is proportional to the radiation received. Ion chambers are the most robust type of dosimeter used for the measurement of absolute dose. Its response is stable with respect to dose rate.

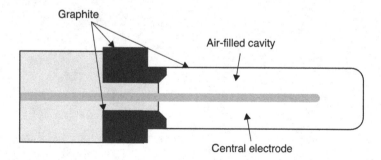

Graphite

Air-filled cavity

Central electrode

Answer 6

The bias voltage is chosen such that the ion pairs produced by the direct ionization move fast enough toward the poles so that there is no significant recombination, yet small enough so that no extra electron–ion pairs are produced due to their acceleration. Usually the bias voltage is between 150 and 300 V.

Question 7
Why must build-up caps be used for high-energy dose measurements with ion chambers?

Question 8
What is the difference between a sealed and open ion chambers?

Question 9
What is a parallel plate ion chamber?

Question 10
What is an extrapolation ion chamber used for?

Question 11
How does a thermoluminescent dosimeter (TLD) work?

Answer 7

The wall thickness of an ion chamber must be greater than or equal to the range of secondary charged particles (ie, electrons), which are produced in the wall. This condition is necessary to provide electronic equilibrium within the sensitive volume of the chamber. In high-energy beams, this condition is not satisfied and a build-up cap is required to add additional thickness to the chamber wall to maintain the condition of electronic equilibrium.

Answer 8

The air chamber cavity can be sealed or open to the atmosphere. The amount of air inside (air mass) an open ion chamber depends on the temperature and pressure of the atmosphere at the point of measurement, therefore when making dose measurement, the charge reading must be corrected for the temperature and pressure. Sealed ion chambers provide a constant response, unaffected by changes in external temperature and pressure, but are vulnerable to leaks.

Answer 9

A parallel plate ion chamber also has a cylindrical collection volume, but its height is much smaller than its radius. This allows the chamber to measure a large volume, but over a narrow depth. They are commonly used for measuring dose close to the surface of a phantom or in the build-up region, and for electrons which have steep dose changes as a function of depth.

Answer 10

Ion chambers have finite spatial extent which makes it difficult to measure dose in superficial layers of a medium (eg, surface dose). Extrapolation ion chambers contain micrometer screws that are used to adjust the spacing between their electrodes. Dose at 0 cm spacing can be extrapolated from a series of measurements taken at progressively smaller spacing. Extrapolation chambers were originally designed for electron dosimetry.

Answer 11

A TLD is made of semiconductor materials that when exposed to ionizing radiation allow electrons to be trapped in metastable states. When heated, these electrons drop into the ground state and light is released. The amount of light released by the material is then proportional to the radiation dose. After heating (annealing), the TLD can be reused.

Question 12
What materials are used in thermoluminescent dosimeters (TLDs)?

Question 13
What is the expected accuracy of a thermoluminescent dosimeter (TLD)?

Question 14
Does the thermoluminescent dosimeter (TLD) accuracy change over time?

Question 15
What is an optically stimulated luminescence detector (OSLD)?

Question 16
What are the advantages of a thermoluminescent dosimeter (TLD) when compared to a optically stimulated luminescence detector (OSLD)?

Question 17
What is the disadvantage of thermoluminescent dosimeters (TLDs) when compared to optically stimulated luminescence detectors (OSLDs)?

Answer 12

Common TLD materials include LiF:Mg, Ti; LiF:Mg,Cu, P; $Li_2B_4O_7$:Mn; $CaSO_4$:Dy; and $CaSO_4$:Mn. LiF:Mg is the most common type of TLD. It is available in a variety of forms, including powder, cards, ribbons, and Teflon chips. It has a physical density (2.64 g/cm³) and effective atomic number (Z_{eff} = 8.2), close to that of tissue (7.4). The lithium used can be Li^6 or Li^7. Li^6 is sensitive to neutrons, Li^7 is not. They can be used in combination to determine the neutron component of the dose. Both $CaSO_4$-based TLD materials have the same density (2.61 g/cm³) and effective atomic number (Z_{eff} = 15.3).

Answer 13

TLDs are an example of a clinically useful secondary dosimeter based on the process of thermoluminescence. They are accurate to within approximately 3% to 5%.

Answer 14

The lowest energy traps release their electrons in less than 10 hours, and so TLDs are typically read 24 hours after the exposure to avoid measuring the light from these electrons. After this period, the accuracy of the TLD is typically maintained if the TLDs are read within about 12 weeks from exposure.

Answer 15

An OSLD is similar to a thermoluminescent dosimeter (TLD) in that radiation of the OSLD causes electrons to move into metastable states. Instead of heating the OSLD to cause the electrons to drop back to the ground state, the material is exposed to a green laser light. The blue light emitted by the descending electrons is proportional to the radiation absorbed by the OSLD. The advantage over TLD is that the OSLD only releases 0.2% of the trapped electron, so it can be reread if necessary. Al_2O_3 is the most common OSL material.

Answer 16

A TLD is smaller than an OSLD, and TLDs have a smaller angular dependence than OSLDs (ie, response to the angle that the radiation enters the dosimeter).

Answer 17

The reading process for TLDs is more time consuming and dose readings from the TLDs are not instantaneous. TLDs typically require 24 hours before being read out. OSLDs can be read out instantaneously.

Question 18

How does a diode detector work?

Question 19

What are the advantages of diodes when compared to the ionization chamber?

Question 20

What are the disadvantages of diodes when compared to the ionization chamber?

Question 21

What factors affect the reading of a diode?

Question 22

When a diode is used for in vivo dose measurement, what dose is the dosimeter reporting?

Question 23

According to TG 51, what dosimeters are used for the calibration of megavoltage linear accelerators?

Question 24

What dosimeter is most often used to find a missing I-125 seed in brachytherapy?

Answer 18

Diodes are semiconductor material. In the depletion layer of the p–n junction there is a natural electric field. When direct ionization radiation hits this region, electron–hole pairs are created. The electrons and holes move in opposite directions under the influence of the natural bias voltage. The charge thus collected is proportional to the dose.

Answer 19

Compared with ion chambers, diode detectors are much more sensitive detectors because of the high density of the material (relative to air) and small amount of energy required to make an electron–hole pair (~2 eV) than to make an electron–ion pair in air (~33 eV). Therefore, they can be made much smaller. Furthermore, diode detectors do not require an external bias voltage.

Answer 20

Compared to the ionization chambers, diodes are energy dependent and its measurement accuracy decreases when the accumulative exposure increases.

Answer 21

A diode detector's sensitivity depends on the dose rate, energy spectrum of the beam, the direction the radiation enters the detector, and the exposure history of the detector. To use the detector for absolute dose measurement, the detector must be calibrated against an ion chamber.

Answer 22

A diode is typically calibrated to the nominal maximum depth of the beam energy. With a build-up cap, the reported dose is typically the dose at d_{max}.

Answer 23

Only ion chambers can be used for absolute calibration of a linear accelerator.

Answer 24

Since the dose rate of an individual seed is very small, a Geiger-Müller detector is best suited for this purpose because of its high sensitivity.

Question 25
What dosimeters are most often used for in vivo measurements?

Question 26
What dosimeters can be used for radioactive isotope leakage measurements?

Question 27
Why is a Geiger counter not an acceptable dosimeter for measurements of linear accelerator (linac) radiation?

Question 28
What types of dosimeters are commonly used for radiation worker exposure monitoring?

Question 29
What dosimeters are used for the relative distribution of dose?

Question 30
How can radiographic film be used for dosimetry?

Answer 25

Diodes, thermoluminescent dosimeters (TLDs), metal–oxide semiconductor field-effect transistors (MOSFETS), and optically stimulated luminescence detector (OSLD) are most often used for in vivo dose measurement.

Diode dosimeters have real-time readouts and are convenient for daily use. They also have the advantage that they do not need a bias voltage and so are safe to put on patients. Ion chambers are not often used because of the concern of the high bias voltage (300 V) that is needed. TLDs and OSLDs do not have real-time readouts. However, multiple detectors can be used at the same time for multiple point dose measurements and later readout.

Answer 26

Isotope leakage measurements require extremely high sensitivity; therefore, a well counter is ideal for this task.

Answer 27

Geiger counters have a period of insensitivity after each burst of radiation called dead time. Linacs work in a pulsed mode, so using a Geiger counter may miss pulses, or it may be completely nonresponsive because of the high dose rate involved.

Answer 28

Radiation badges or rings required to measure radiation worker exposure typically contain film, thermoluminescent dosimeter (TLD), or optically stimulated luminescence detector (OSLD).

Answer 29

Film is best for measurement of relative dose distribution. Ion chamber or diode arrays can also be used, but have much lower resolution.

Answer 30

On exposure to a radiation field, radiographic film undergoes chemical changes in silver bromide crystals which cause the formation of a latent image. Development and fixation processes remove undeveloped crystal granules leaving dark regions where the radiation has exposed the film. The opacity of these areas depends on the quantity of absorbed energy. A densitometer is used to quantify the optical density of regions of the film. The optical density can be used to quantify dose through the use of the Hurter and Driffield (H&D) curve.

Question 31

What are the advantages and disadvantages of using radiographic film for dosimetry?

Question 32

How is radiochromic film different from radiographic film?

Question 33

In determining dose using a Fricke ferrous sulfate dosimeter, what does the quantity G represent?

Question 34

What dosimeters are used for measurement of neutron dose?

Question 35

According to TG 51, how often do the ion chambers need to be calibrated. Who is qualified to do the calibration? What does the calibration agency provide?

Answer 31

Advantages: High spatial resolution and low cost.

Disadvantages: Must be calibrated against an ion chamber. Film displays significant energy dependence. Air pockets can cause artifacts when films are placed in phantoms. Correction factors may be required for exposures in the nonlinear region of the Hurter and Driffield (H&D) curve. Low-energy scattered photons interact strongly in film via the photoelectric effect due to the presence of silver, which has a relatively high-Z compared to soft tissue and bone. Additional uncertainties are introduced by differences in emulsions and processing conditions. It also requires chemical processing.

Answer 32

Radiographic film density is achieved via chemical changes in silver bromide crystals. However, in radiochromic film, density is achieved through a polymerization process. Unlike radiographic film, radiochromic film does not require chemical processing.

Both types of film dosimetry require the measurement of optical density. In radiographic film, optical density is measured using a densitometer. Measurement of optical density for radiochromic film requires the use of a spectrophotometer, microdensitometer, or laser scanner. Radiochromic film is also approximately tissue equivalent (radiographic film is not as it contains silver) and has low energy dependence, a large dynamic range, and is not sensitive in the visible spectrum.

Answer 33

Fricke ferrous sulfate dosimeters make use of an oxidation reaction which converts ferrous ions to ferric ions. The concentration of ferric ions is related to the dose absorbed. G represents the radiation chemical yield (number of ferric ions produced per 100 eV).

Answer 34

Tissue-equivalent proportional counters (TEPCs), superheated drop, Bonner spheres, neutron monitoring film, type A (NTA film), fission track, and thermoluminescent dosimeter (TLD) albedo detectors can all be used for neutron dosimetry.

Answer 35

Ion chambers must be calibrated when first purchased, after being repaired, when a problem is detected, and at least every two years. This is performed by an Accredited Dosimetry Calibration Laboratory (ADCL), whose calibrations are directly traceable to the National Institute of Standards and Technology (NIST). The calibration lab provides the absorbed dose to water calibration coefficient for the ion chamber being used. This calibration is termed "directly traceable" to NIST. A chamber can be cross calibrated by a physicist to a directly traceable chamber, and would then be "indirectly traceable."

Question 36
How do metal–oxide semiconductor field-effect transistors (MOSFETs) work as radiation dosimeters?

Question 37
What are advantages and disadvantages of metal–oxide semiconductor field-effect transistors (MOSFETs) when compared to thermoluminescent dosimeters (TLDs)?

Question 38
What special problems do the calibration of small fields, such as fields used in stereotactic radiosurgery (SRS) and stereotactic body radiation therapy (SBRT), present?

Question 39
What device is used to measure optical density in film dosimetry?

Question 40
What is the optical density of a film if 7% of light is transmitted through it?

Answer 36

MOSFET is an acronym which stands for metal–oxide semiconductor field-effect transistor. There are four main components to a MOSFET: a drain, a source, a gate, and a bulk substrate. In a p-channel MOSFET, a negative voltage is applied to the gate which causes a buildup of holes in the underlying substrate. When a sufficiently large voltage is applied to the gate there will be enough holes in the substrate to allow current to flow between the source and the drain. The voltage at which current is able to flow is known as the threshold voltage. Ionizing radiation interacts to create electron holes. The presence of holes causes a measurable change in the threshold voltage which is proportional to the dose.

Answer 37

The major advantage is that dose readings from MOSFETs are instantaneous. The disadvantages of MOSFETs are that they are not water equivalent and have angular dependence.

Answer 38

Loss of charged particle equilibrium, detector noise, partial occlusion of the radiation source, and perturbation of the radiation field by the detector itself are all concerns in small field dosimetry. Purpose built microchambers or diodes should be used.

Answer 39

A densitometer or calibrated film scanner.

Answer 40

Since optical density $OD = \log_{10} \frac{I_0}{I_t}$, where I_0 is the incident light intensity and I_t is the transmitted light intensity, we have

$$I_t = 0.07 I_0 \Rightarrow OD \ \log_{10}\left(\frac{1}{0.07}\right) = 1.15$$

5

PHOTON TREATMENT

MATTHEW C. WARD AND SALIM BALIK

Question 1

Explain the concept of "beam quality." What is one simple way of defining "beam quality"?

Question 2

Explain the concept of "beam hardening." After a beam passes through a filter, how do the maximum energy, average energy, half-value layer (HVL), and dose rate change?

Question 3

Explain the relationship of tube voltage, tube current, and filament current to the relative output of a kV diagnostic X-ray tube.

Turn page to see the answers.   115

Answer 1

Beam quality describes the energy spectrum of an X-ray (or Gamma-ray) photon beam. Some photon beams, for example, Co-60, are nearly monoenergetic [1.25 megaelectron volt (MeV) average]. Other beams, for example, a 6 MV linac beam, are poly-energetic. MeV implies one energy whereas the 6 MV implies a spectrum, with 6 MeV as the maximum energy. The beam quality from each manufacturer and machine is slightly different for beams with the same nominal energy. For therapy photon beams, the detailed beam quality is measured by a curve called the percent depth dose (PDD) curve. The PDD value at 10 cm depth is often used to report the quality of the beam in one number. For diagnostic beams, the kVp or half-value layer is used to define the beam quality instead of PDD.

Answer 2

Beam hardening occurs when the beam passes through any matter, which acts as a filter, absorbing low-energy photons. The transmitted beam will have an increased average energy, decreased dose rate while the maximum energy is unchanged. For a diagnostic beam, this increase in energy results in an increase in HVL. In the figure, the black spectrum is the initial beam and the gray is the filtered beam.

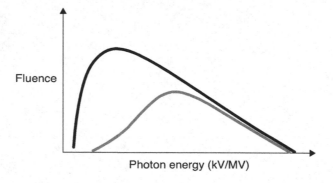

Answer 3

The output in a kV X-ray tube is proportional to the tube current, the square of the tube voltage, and exponentially with the filament current.

Question 4
Why is Cerrobend employed for custom blocking? What is the transmission through a block?

Question 5
How many half-value layers (HVLs) of the Cerrobend are necessary to limit the transmission to 10% and 1%?

Question 6
How does a physical wedge affect beam quality?

Question 7
Does a virtual wedge affect the beam quality?

Answer 4

Cerrobend is an alloy of bismuth, lead, tin, and cadmium. It is useful as a high density (9.4 g/cm³) and high-Z material with a low melting point to quickly create a block in a desired shape. The goal is to achieve ≤5% primary beam transmission which means 4.3 half value layers of cerrobend or more.

Answer 5

3.322 HVLs are necessary to limit the dose to 10% transmission. 6.644 HVLs are necessary for 1% transmission. As you can see, $3.322 \left(\frac{1}{2}^{3.322} = 10\% \right)$ is a useful number to remember to quickly calculate exponential decay as applied to either radioactive decay or transmission through HVLs.

Answer 6

A physical wedge, comprised of a triangle-shaped metal material that generates a gradient of beam intensities at depth. This differentially filters the low-energy X-rays, leading to beam hardening. The degree of beam hardening is more pronounced near the thicker "heel" of the wedge. A physical wedge is also responsible for increased scatter.

Answer 7

A virtual wedge does not produce variable beam hardening as the gradient profile is created by slowly opening one collimator jaw of the linear accelerator, rather than transmission through a physical wedge. Any scatter from the jaw is reduced by shielding in the head of the machine and does not contribute significantly to the dose experienced by the patient.

Question 8

Describe the spatial distribution of photons generated by bremsstrahlung. How is the distribution affected by the energy of the incident electron?

Question 9

What is a Thoraeus filter?

Question 10

Why is the order of layers in the Thoraeus filter important?

Question 11

What are bremsstrahlung interactions and why do they happen?

Answer 8

For kV incident electron energies, the X-rays are produced isotropically (in all directions). With megavolt (MV) incident electron energies, the X-ray distribution becomes progressively more aligned with the direction of the incident electrons. Therefore, a kV X-ray tube may use a reflection target where useful X-rays are at 90° to the electron beam, whereas an MV linear accelerator uses a transmission target.

Answer 9

A Thoraeus filter is commonly used with diagnostic X-ray tubes. The filter consists of tin, copper, and aluminum layers to remove low-energy photons and characteristic X-rays from the beam. These low-energy photons do not contribute to image quality but increase patient dose.

Answer 10

The order of filter layers is important because tin contributes the most to filtration of the characteristic X-rays of the tungsten target, which fall between 58 and 69 keV. Tin's characteristic X-rays are of very low energy and can be filtered with copper. Copper's characteristic X-rays are filtered by a thin film of aluminum, leading to a hard beam capable of producing sharp images.

Answer 11

Bremsstrahlung interactions occur when a high-energy electron pass near the nucleus of an atom. The electron is deflected by the nucleus due to its Coulomb force. The electron undergoes sudden acceleration in a different direction, losing all or part of its energy in the process, which is converted into a photon. A single electron may undergo multiple bremsstrahlung interactions before finally coming to rest.

Question 12
What is the most probable energy of a 10 MV photon beam?

Question 13
Describe the source of and difference between inherent and added filtration.

Question 14
How is beam penumbra defined?

Question 15
What are the three main sources of beam penumbra in therapy photon beams?

Answer 12

High-energy photon beams are created by bremsstrahlung interactions and therefore contain a spectrum of energies. The most probable energy is approximately one third that of the maximum energy, which by convention is used to name the beam. Therefore, for a 10 MV beam the maximum energy is 10 MeV and the most probable energy is approximately 3.33 MeV. This is not the same as the average energy, which is more difficult to calculate.

Answer 13

Inherent filtration in a linear accelerator is typically caused by the tungsten target itself—as electrons interact with the target, a spectrum of photons are created via bremsstrahlung interactions. The low-energy photons may interact and be absorbed by the remaining tungsten before emerging as a part of the spectrum. This effect increases as the thickness of the target increases. Added filtration is intentionally placed in the path of a beam with the goal of increasing the average beam energy (beam hardening) or decreasing the intensity of a beam.

Answer 14

Beam penumbra (umbra is Latin for "shadow") is the gradual reduction of beam intensity at the edge of a photon field. It is typically measured as the width between the 80% and 20% isodose lines, although 90% to 10% isodose lines are also used.

Answer 15

The three main sources of beam penumbra are transmission penumbra, geometric penumbra, and internal penumbra. Transmission penumbra occurs as the beam passes through the edge of the jaw, block, or multileaf collimator (MLC). Geometric penumbra occurs because the source is not a point-source. Internal penumbra is due to scatter within the patient.

Question 16

Is there a difference between the first and second half-value layer (HVL) for a cobalt unit? What about a diagnostic X-ray tube?

Question 17

How is the beam energy changed by the flattening filter?

Question 18

How is the beam flatness specified?

Answer 16

Cobalt-60 generates a near-monoenergetic beam (1.17 MeV, 1.32 MeV combined for an average of 1.25 MeV) and therefore the $HVL_1 = HVL_2 = HVL_3$. However, diagnostic tubes use bremsstrahlung X-ray generation to produce a spectrum of energies. After the beam passes through the first HVL, due to the concept of "beam hardening," the second HVL is now greater than the first.

Answer 17

X-ray intensity is forward peaked after the target before the flattening filter. The flattening filter is thicker in the middle and tapers off toward the edges so that the central region is attenuated more than the periphery to make the beam flat. As a result, the beam will be hardened more in the center than the periphery (lower average energy in the periphery). This results in a beam that is peaked at depths greater than 10 cm. The flattening filter also reduces the dose rate significantly.

Answer 18

Beam flatness is specified at 10 cm depth and within the area bounded by 80% of the field size or 1 cm inside the field edge. The beam flatness should be within ±3% of the central axis dose at 10 cm depth.

Question 19

How does a wedge filter change the isodose lines? What is wedge angle?

Question 20

Parallel opposed beams are frequently used in radiation therapy. They provide uniform dose distribution for the target with a simple and reproducible setup. One disadvantage of this technique is called "tissue lateral effect." How does this effect change with energy and patient thickness?

Question 21

How is "integral dose" defined and how does it change with energy?

Answer 19

The wedge tilts the isodose lines toward its thin edge. The angle between central axis and the isodose lines at 10 cm depth is the wedge angle.

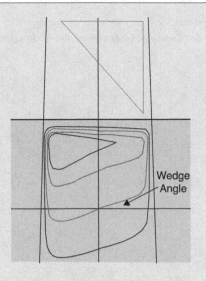

Wedge Angle

Answer 20

The midpoint between the opposed beams is the prescription point. The maximum dose to the midpoint dose (prescription point) ratio increases with patient thickness and decreases with energy. As a result, it is better to use higher energy X-ray beams (>10 MV) for large patients (>20 cm) to improve homogeneity of the dose distribution and preserve subcutaneous tissue.

Answer 21

Integral dose is simply mass × dose if dose is uniform throughout the region, or the sum of the energy deposited. If dose volume histogram is calculated, the integral dose is the area under the contour of the external, which includes all tissue of the patient. The unit of "integral dose" is kg/Gy or joule. It is used in determining treatment plan quality in regards to how much dose is delivered outside the target. The integral dose decreases with energy.

Question 22

What are the advantages and disadvantages of a flattening filter free (FFF) linear accelerator?

Question 23

Define the term "effective energy" for a heterogeneous X-ray beam.

Question 24

What term is used to specify the quality of a megavoltage X-ray beam?

Question 25

Why are electron energies written as megaelectron volts (MeVs) but photon energies as megavolts (MVs)?

Answer 22

New linear accelerators (linacs) are available with an FFF design. Linacs require a flattening filter to produce flat beams across large open fields. However, the flattening filter lowers the dose rate of the machine and produces beam hardening. With small-field intensity modulated radiation therapy (IMRT) treatments, the multileaf collimators (MLCs) are used to deliberately modulate the intensity of the beam. For these treatments, the filter is no longer required. The advantages of this approach include a significantly increased dose rate (>1,000 MU/min versus 300 to 600 MU/min) and decreased variation in energy spectrum (due to beam hardening). The disadvantages of this approach include a possible increase in skin dose (less beam hardening) and the inability to treat large, flat, open fields without the use of the MLCs. Some manufactures add a thin filter to remove very low-energy photons for nonflat beams.

Answer 23

The "effective energy" is defined as the energy of a monoenergetic X-ray beam that has the same half-value layer as the heterogeneous X-ray beam.

Answer 24

The percent depth dose (PDD) value at 10 cm depth of a 10 cm × 10 cm field size with source to skin distance of 100 cm is used to define the beam quality.

Answer 25

Electron energies are monoenergetic as they leave the accelerating waveguide but photons are heterogeneous in energy. MV photon energy represents the highest energy X-ray (in MeVs) in the spectrum.

Question 1

5.2 FACTORS AFFECTING PHOTON DOSE DEPOSITION

What is the definition of percent depth dose (PDD) for a given field size?

Question 2

How and why is the percent depth dose (PDD) at 10 cm affected by increases in field size, energy, source to skin distance (SSD), and physical wedges?

Question 3

Explain the shape of a megavoltage central-axis percent depth dose (PDD) curve. Graph the PDD curve of a 6 MV beam. Label the curve at 0, 1.5, and 10 cm depth. Label the approximate slope of the beam between 1.5 and 10 cm?

Answer 1

For a given field size, PDD (expressed in percentage) is measured along the central axis and defined as the ratio of a dose at a given depth d to the dose at a reference depth (usually d_{max}) on the central axis.

$$\%DD = \frac{\text{Dose at depth } d}{\text{Dose at ref depth } (d_{max})} \times 100\%$$

Answer 2

	PDD	Why?
Field size	Increases	Increased scatter
Energy	Increases	Increased penetration due to increased energy
SSD	Increases	Inverse square law (Mayneord factor)
Physical wedge	Increases	Beam hardening

Answer 3

The PDD curve reports dose deposition as a function of depth for a radiation beam. The PDD on the surface for megavoltage energies is below 100% as the incident photons produce high-energy electrons which travel a distance before coming to rest and depositing energy. This effect explains the "skin sparing" properties of megavoltage therapy. The peak in the curve known as D_{max}, occurs deeper. The curve then declines, or attenuates, due to a combination of the inverse-square law, absorption, and scatter.

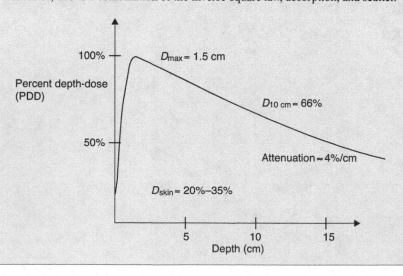

Question 4

What is the typical d_{max} for cobalt-60 (Co-60), 6, 10, 15, and 18 MV beams using a 10 cm × 10 cm field size?

Question 5

What is the percent change in the percent depth dose (PDD) per centimeter for cobalt-60 (Co-60), 6 and 10 MV photons under standard conditions?

Question 6

While you are on-call over the weekend you wish to treat a 20 cm long by 8 cm wide posterior to anterior (PA) spine field. Calculate the equivalent square necessary to complete the hand calculation. Why is the equivalent square necessary?

Answer 4

The d_{max} is slightly different for every machine and beam; however, typical values are 0.5, 1.5, 2.5, 3.0, and 3.2 to 3.5 cm for each energy, respectively.

Answer 5

Co-60 attenuates at approximately 4% per cm, 6 MV beams attenuate at approximately 3.5% per cm, and 10 MV attenuates at approximately 3.3% per cm. Note that these numbers are approximation, as the values change with depth.

Answer 6

$$S = \frac{4A}{P}$$

where S is side of equivalent square, A and P are, respectively, the area and perimeter of the rectangular field.

$$\frac{4A}{P} = \frac{4 \times 20 \times 8}{2 \times (20 + 8)} = \frac{640}{56}$$

$$S = 11.4 \text{ cm}$$

The square field with 11.4 cm side is equivalent to a 20 cm × 8 cm rectangular field. Usually percent depth dose (PDD) or tissue maximum ratio (TMR) values are only tabulated for square fields. A rectangular field will have approximately the same PDD or TMR as its equivalent square field. There are also other more complex methods to approximate the PDD or TMR for irregular field shapes like Clarkson's method.

Question 7

Percent depth dose (PDD) values are generally tabulated for source to skin distance (SSD) of 100 cm. How can we estimate PDDs for SSDs other than 100 cm? What is the limitation of this technique?

Question 8

Using the inverse square law, derive the Mayneord F factor.

Question 9

The percent depth dose (PDD) for a 6 MV beam with a 12 cm × 12 cm field size at 11 cm depth and 100 cm source to skin distance (SSD) is 64.7%. Estimate the PDD for the same field if the SSD is increased to 115 cm.

Answer 7

The Mayneord F factor is used to estimate PDDs for different SSDs. The F factor is an estimation of PDD changes based solely on the inverse-square law. It assumes that the amount of scatter is constant as SSD changes, which is not quite correct and limits the accuracy of this method. For low energies, tissue-to-air ratio (TAR) correction to Mayneord F factor method can be used if TAR tables are available.

Answer 8

Understanding the derivation will help you remember the F-factor equation and how it is used. Knowing the simple inverse-square relationship is all that the F factor is based on.
First, the F factor is defined simply as follows:

$$F = \frac{PDD_2}{PDD_1}$$

Since percent depth dose (PDD) increases with increasing source to skin distance (SSD), note already that by definition the F factor is greater than 1 for increasing PDD values. Now, applying the definition of PDD:

$$F = \frac{PDD_2}{PDD_1} = \frac{\left(\dfrac{D_2}{D_{max}}\right)}{\left(\dfrac{D_1}{D_{max}}\right)}$$

Applying the inverse-square relationship we obtain:

$$F = \frac{\left(\dfrac{SSD_2 + d_{max}}{SSD_2 + d}\right)^2}{\left(\dfrac{SSD_1 + d_{max}}{SSD_1 + d}\right)^2}$$

Finally, a little algebra gives us the format we see most commonly in books:

$$F = \left(\frac{SSD_1 + d}{SSD_2 + d} \times \frac{SSD_2 + d_{max}}{SSD_1 + d_{max}}\right)^2$$

Answer 9

This question requires the use of the Mayneord F factor. This method uses the inverse-square law to estimate the change in PDD due to a change in SSD. It does not account for changes in scatter which is typically ignored due to its relatively small contribution in the change in PDD. In this equation, d is the depth in tissue, r is the field size, and f is the SSD.

$$F = \left(\frac{PDD_2(d, r, f_2)}{PDD_1(d, r, f_1)}\right) = \left(\frac{SSD_1 + d}{SSD_2 + d} \times \frac{SSD_2 + d_{max}}{SSD_1 + d_{max}}\right)^2$$

$$F = \left(\frac{100 + 11}{115 + 11} \times \frac{115 + 1.5}{100 + 1.5}\right)^2$$

$$F = 1.011$$

$$PDD(115\ cm) = PDD(100\ cm) \times 1.011 = 65.4\%$$

Remember that for a larger source to skin distance (SSD), the F factor is above one and the PDD will be greater.

Question 10
Approximate the dose delivered to 1.5 cm if 100 cGy is delivered to a point at 10 cm depth using a 6 MV beam with a field size of 10 cm × 10 cm.

Question 11
By convention, where is field size defined?

Question 12
Why are high-energy photons (>10 MV) generally not recommended in the treatment of lung cancer?

Answer 10

Knowing that for a 6 MV beam and a 10 cm × 10 cm field size, d_{max} is approximately 1.5 cm and 67% of the D_{max} is delivered to 10 cm. Therefore, $D(10\ cm) = PDD(10\ cm) \times D_{max}$ and $D(d_{max}) = 149$ cGy.

Answer 11

Field size is typically defined at machine isocenter, 100 cm from the source. This would then be on the patient surface for source to skin distance setup, or at isocenter for source to axis distance (SAD) setup.

Answer 12

The difference in electron density between lung and the soft tissue/bone of the chest wall presents special problems in the management of lung cancer. High-energy photons can contribute to increased scatter dosing in the lung. Also, the larger buildup region of high-energy photons may compromise tumor coverage at its periphery.

Question 13

What is the "buildup region" and why does it occur? How does the buildup region depend on the energy of a photon?

Question 14

How does depth of maximum dose (d_{max}) vary as a function of field size? Why?

Question 15

Why does percent depth dose (PDD) increase with field size?

Answer 13

The buildup region is the initial region on the percent depth dose (PDD) curve between the surface of the patient and d_{max}. Remember that dose deposition of photons is dependent on secondary electrons. While the photons are steadily attenuated exponentially as a function of the inverse-square law, high-energy photons require some depth in tissue to generate secondary electrons, thus explaining why the deposited dose is low at the surface of the irradiated tissue.

Answer 14

The depth of d_{max} slightly decreases as a function of field size. For example, a d_{max} of 1.5 cm is estimated for a 6 MV photon and a 10 cm × 10 cm field, whereas a 20 cm × 20 cm field would expect to show a d_{max} of 1.4 cm. This is due to increased scatter contributing to superficial dose deposition, bringing d_{max} closer to the surface.

Answer 15

PDD increases as field size increases due to scatter from the off-axis tissue. Note that both primary dose (photons emitted directly from the linac head) and secondary dose (scatter from surrounding tissue) contribute to PDD. Although both the dose at depth (D_d) and the dose at d_{max} rise, the D_d rises more than the dose at d_{max} (D_{max}), therefore PDD increases.

Question 16
How does the percent depth dose (PDD) field size dependence change with energy?

Question 17
Explain the difference between and advantages of monitor unit (MU) calculation using tissue maximum ratio (TMR; source to axis distance [SAD] technique) compared to a percent depth dose (PDD; source to skin distance [SSD] technique).

Question 18
Draw a diagram defining the tissue-to-air ratio (TAR). Explain the effect field size and beam energy has on the TAR?

Answer 16

The increase in PDD with field size is larger for low energies. With higher energies, scatter is mostly in the direction of the photon, thus lateral scatter is less.

Answer 17

PDD calculations are convenient when the SSD does not change and SSD is at the standard calibration distance of 100 cm. However, for a multifield treatment SSDs will typically vary or the patient will have to be moved for each beam. The TMR method is independent of SSD and has an advantage in this situation.

Answer 18

The TAR is defined as the dose at a point in tissue divided by the dose in air at the same distance from the source. Because the distance from the source is in both the numerator and denominator, the TAR does not vary with source to skin distance (SSD), giving a key advantage for calculations with a variable SSD; multifield source to axis distance (SAD) setup. If the field enlarges (with a constant depth), there is more scatter in the tissue (numerator). However, there is no scatter in air and the denominator remains constant, therefore the TAR increases. Since higher energies are more penetrating in tissue, the TAR increases with increasing energy.

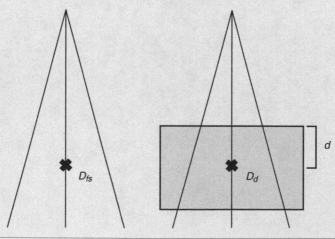

Question 19

Define and show the relationship between percent depth dose (PDD), tissue-to-air ratio (TAR), inverse-square law (ISL), and peak scatter factor (PSF) on a diagram?

Question 20

What is the relationship between the peak scatter factor (PSF) and the backscatter factor (BSF)?

Question 21

What is the approximate peak scatter factor (PSF) for high-energy (≥6 MV) photon beams?

Answer 19

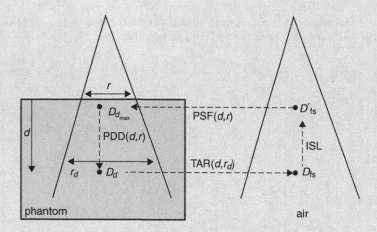

We can convert the dose at these four locations shown in the figure by TAR, PDD, ISL, and PSF. Let f represent the source to skin distance.

$$D_d = \frac{\text{PDD}(f,d,r) \times D_{d_{max}}}{100}$$

$$D_{fs} = \frac{D_d}{\text{TAR}(d,r_d)}$$

$$D'_{fs} = \sqrt{D_{fs}^2 \left(\frac{f}{f+d}\right)^2}$$

$$D_{d_{max}} = \text{PSF}(r) \times D'_{fs}$$

Note that the peak scatter factor is a special case of the TAR and is defined only at d_{max} whereas TAR could be at any depth.

Answer 20

The BSF is the special case of PSF when low-energy photons with a d_{max} of zero are considered. If d_{max} is close to zero, the only scatter in tissue contributing to the dose to d_{max} is backward, hence the name "backscatter."

Answer 21

Since high-energy photons tend to scatter forward the PSF decreases to only a few percent for higher energy beams (PSF between 1.05 and 1.1). The PSF (or more precisely, the backscatter factor) is greater for low-energy photons due to increased lateral scatter in tissue (could be as high as 40% to 50% for diagnostic X-rays).

Question 22
Define tissue maximum ratio (TMR). How does it relate to tissue-to-air ratio (TAR)?

Question 23
Both the definition of percent depth dose (PDD) and tissue maximum ratio (TMR) could be written as $D_d/D_{d_{max}}$. Why are they different?

Question 24
You plan to treat a 10 cm × 10 cm tumor in a large patient with a single 6 MV field. Rather than the classic source to skin distance (SSD) setup, you choose a source to axis distance (SAD) setup and place the isocenter in the target a depth of 10 cm from the surface and prescribe 10 Gy in a single fraction. The patient is delayed after simulation and returns three weeks later, having lost 40 lbs. From a new CT you measure the new depth to be 8 cm. Explain two methods of calculating the new dose to the isocenter given the same SAD.

Answer 22

$$TMR = \frac{\text{Dose at depth } d}{\text{Dose at } d_{max}}$$

Note that both doses are calculated using the same source to point distance (ie, source to axis distance [SAD]). TMR is related to TAR by the peak scatter factor (PSF) (derivation not shown):

$$TMR = \frac{TAR}{PSF}$$

Answer 23

PDD is calculated using the same source to skin distance (SSD) and different depths, TMR is calculated using the same source to axis distance (SAD) and therefore is independent of SSD.

Answer 24

This is an example that takes advantage of tissue maximum ratio (TMR) calculations. Since the source to skin distance (SSD) has now changed, using a percent depth dose (PDD) approach would require a Mayneord calculation. The TMR approach is independent of the SSD and requires only the depth in tissue to calculate, assuming the field size (defined at depth) has not changed. TMR can be found in a table. Using the appropriate values as follows, the new dose to the isocenter is 10.75 Gy:

$$\frac{D_{d1}(\text{SAD, Field Size})}{D_{d2}(\text{SAD, Field Size})} = \frac{D_{8 \text{ cm}}(100 \text{ cm, } 10 \text{ cm})}{D_{10 \text{ cm}}(100 \text{ cm, } 10 \text{ cm})} = \frac{TMR(8 \text{ cm})}{TMR(10 \text{ cm})} = \frac{0.841}{0.782} = 1.075$$

Question 25

The tissue maximum ratios (TMR) of a 5 cm × 5 cm field size 16 MV beam source at 8 and 10 cm depth are 0.80 and 0.75, respectively. An oddly shaped square patient made of water has an anterior to posterior/posterior to anterior (AP/PA) diameter of 16 cm and a lateral diameter of 20 cm at the isocenter placed in the center of the patient. What is the maximum dose outside the target area if a four-field box approach is used to treat a single fraction of 2 Gy to the isocenter and with equal weights from each beam of 5 cm × 5 cm size?

Question 26

A patient's surface can be irregular depending on the site that we are treating. However, it is often desirable to have a uniform dose distribution. How are the surface irregularities managed during radiation therapy? Discuss advantages and disadvantages of all methods.

Answer 25

This question illustrates the value of the TMR. For a single isocenter setup, the contribution from each beam will be even at 0.5 Gy. The actual d_{max} is not necessary information and will be the location of the hot spot. Realizing that the largest hot spot for one field would be at the deepest prescription depth, we can calculate this using the TMR definition.

$$TMR = \frac{D_{depth}(SAD, \text{ Field Size})}{D_{d_{max}}(SAD, \text{ Field Size})}$$

$$0.75 = \frac{D_{10\ cm}(100\ cm, \ 5\ cm)}{D_{d_{max}}(100\ cm, \ 5\ cm)} = \frac{0.5\ Gy}{D_{d_{max}}}$$

$$D_{d_{max}} = 0.667\ Gy \ \ (33\% \text{ hot spot})$$

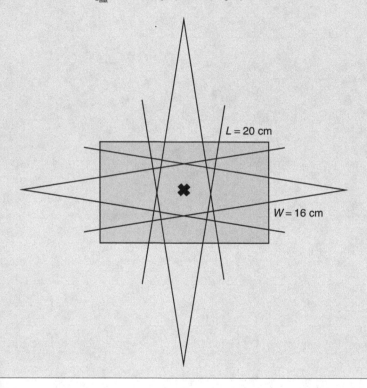

$L = 20$ cm

$W = 16$ cm

Answer 26

A bolus material can be placed on the skin surface to even out the irregularity of the patient surface. Adding a bolus will, however, remove the skin sparing effect of megavoltage radiation. Alternatively, compensators may be used. A compensator filter attenuates the beam in the region of the "missing tissue." Other techniques to manage surface irregularities include using wedge filters or blocking parts of the tissue for some of the fractions of the treatment.

Question 27

For the treatment setup shown in the following figure with a 6 MV treatment photon beam, central axis percent depths dose (PDD) at depths of 10, 12, and 13 cm are 67.8%, 60.9%, and 57.7%, respectively. Calculate the PDD for point P where $h = 3$ cm and $d = 10$ cm using effective source to skin distance (SSD) method, tissue maximum ratio (TMR) ratio method, and isodose shift method (SSD = 100 cm, field size 10 cm × 10 cm, TMR $(10, 11 \times 11) = 0.793$, TMR $(13, 11 \times 11) = 0.710$, isodose shift factor for 6 MV, $k = 0.7$, ref Khan). *Note*: The TMR method gives the most accurate result.

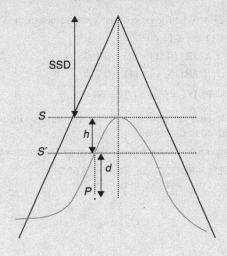

Khan FM. *Khan's The physics of Radiation Therapy*, 4th Edition; 2010 Lippincott Williams & Wilkins, Philadelphia, PA.

Question 28

Which isodose line determines the dosimetric field size?

Answer 27

Effective SSD method: This method is correcting the d_{max} value difference between S and S' planes using the inverse-square law factor:

$$\text{Correction Factor, } CF = \left(\frac{SSD + d_{max}}{SSD + h + d_{max}} \right)^2 = \left(\frac{100 + 1.5}{100 + 3 + 1.5} \right)^2 = 0.94$$

$$PDD_P = 0.94 \times 67.8 = 63.7\%$$

TMR method: In this case, the CF will be the ratio of the TMR values using S and S' as flat patient surface. Field size projected at point P is 11 cm × 11 cm:

$$CF = \frac{TMR(10,\ 11 \times 11)}{TMR(13,\ 11 \times 11)} = \frac{0.793}{0.710} = 1.12$$

$$PDD_P = 57.7 \times 1.12 = 64.4\%$$

Isodose shift method: We need to find the value of PDD for the same isodose lines passing through depth x on central axis and P as illustrated in the following:

$$PDD_x = PDD_P \text{ such that } x + k \times h = 10, \text{ then } x = 12 \text{ where } k = 0.7.$$

$$PDD_P = PDD(12 \text{ cm},\ 10 \times 10) = 60.9\%$$

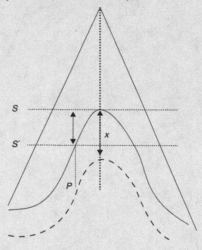

Answer 28

The 50% isodose line defines the field size. The field's size changes with distance due to divergence, and so is defined at the machine isocenter.

Question 29

What is the name of the technique used to calculate dose from irregular fields?

Question 1

5.3 MONITOR UNIT CALCULATIONS

What are "reference conditions" and why are they important? Give an example of common "reference conditions."

Question 2

What two components make up the total dose to tissue at depth?

Question 3

Suppose a 6 MV beam is unconventionally calibrated to deliver 1.5 cGy/MU to d_{max} (1.5 cm) at a source to skin distance (SSD) of 100 cm via a 10 cm × 10 cm field in water. How many monitor units (MUs) would be necessary to deliver 100 cGy to 10 cm via a 10 cm × 10 cm field in water (SSD = 100 cm)?

Answer 29

Clarkson's method. The technique involves dividing an irregular field with blocking into sectors to approximate the scatter from each sector.

Answer 1

Reference conditions are the conditions at which the beam is calibrated. It is critically important to specify these conditions, otherwise systematic errors in dose calculations can occur. One example of common reference conditions is that the beam may be calibrated (per AAPM TG-51) such that 1 monitor unit (MU) is equal to 1 cGy deposited by a 6 MV photon at d_{max} using a 10 cm $\times$ 10 cm field size in water with a source to skin distance (SSD) of 100 cm. Note that field size is determined at 100 cm from the source.

Almond PR, Biggs PJ, Coursey BM, et al. AAPM's TG-51 protocol for clinical reference dosimetry of high-energy photon and electron beams. *Med Phys*. 1999;26(9):1847–1870.

Answer 2

The dose to a point at depth is the sum of the primary dose (dose directly from the head of the machine) and the scattered dose. The scattered dose may come from scatter within the machine or from within the patient.

Answer 3

This is the simplest form of MU calculation:

$$\frac{\text{Dose}}{\text{MU}} \text{ at depth} = \left(\frac{\text{Dose}}{\text{MU}} \text{ at } d_{max} \right) \times \text{PDD}$$

Knowing that the percent depth dose (PDD) at 10 cm of a 6 MV beam is roughly 67%:

$$\frac{\text{Dose}}{\text{MU}} \text{ at depth} = \left(1.5 \ \frac{\text{cGy}}{\text{MU}} \right) \times (0.67) = 1.005 \text{ cGy/MU}$$

$$\text{MU Required} = \frac{100 \text{ cGy}}{1.005 \text{ cGy/MU}} = 99.5 \approx 100 \text{ MU}$$

Question 4

Now suppose a 6 MV beam is even more unconventionally calibrated to deliver 1.5 cGy/MU at 3 cm with a source to skin distance of 100 cm via a 10 cm × 10 cm field in water. Given that the percent depth dose (PDD) at 3 cm of a 6 MV beam is roughly 95%, how many monitor units (MUs) would be necessary to deliver 100 cGy to 10 cm via a 10 cm × 10 cm field in water?

Question 5

Consider a 6 MV beam with a source to skin distance (SSD) of 100 cm and a field size of 10 cm × 10 cm. The physician wishes to prescribe 180 cGy to a depth of 7.0 cm. You know that the dose rate is 0.956 cGy/MU at d_{max} and the percent depth dose at 7.0 cm is 78.2%. How many monitor units (MUs) should be given?

Question 6

Explain the terms S_c and S_p. What are they a function of? What are their typical values?

Answer 4

This is one step more complicated than the previous question (Question 3). Since the dose rate is calibrated at a depth other than d_{max}, we need to correct via the inverse-square law. This is because the definition of PDD is percent of D_{max} ($d_{max} = 1.5$ cm).

$$\frac{\text{Dose}}{\text{MU}} \text{ at depth} = \left(\frac{\text{Dose}}{\text{MU}} \text{ at } d_{max} \right) \times \text{PDD}$$

but

$$\frac{\text{Dose}}{\text{MU}} \text{ at } d_{max} = \left(\frac{\text{Dose}}{\text{MU}} \text{ at depth 3cm} \right) / \text{PDD (3cm)}$$

$$\frac{\text{Dose}}{\text{MU}} \text{ at } d_{max} = \left(1.5 \frac{\text{cGy}}{\text{MU}} \right) / 0.95$$

$$\frac{\text{Dose}}{\text{MU}} \text{ at } d_{max} = 1.58 \frac{\text{cGy}}{\text{MU}}$$

Now, we can use the previous equation along with the PDD given.

$$\frac{\text{Dose}}{\text{MU}} \text{ at depth} = \left(1.58 \frac{\text{cGy}}{\text{MU}} \right) \times 0.67$$

$$\frac{\text{Dose}}{\text{MU}} \text{ at depth} = 1.06 \frac{\text{cGy}}{\text{MU}}$$

So to deliver 100 cGy, we need 106 MU.

Answer 5

$$\frac{\text{Dose}}{\text{MU}} \text{ at depth} = \left(\frac{\text{Dose}}{\text{MU}} \text{ at reference} \right) \times \text{PDD}$$

$$\frac{\text{Dose}}{\text{MU}} \text{ at depth} = \left(0.956 \frac{\text{cGy}}{\text{MU}} \right) \times (0.782)$$

$$\frac{\text{Dose}}{\text{MU}} \text{ at depth} = 0.748 \frac{\text{cGy}}{\text{MU}}$$

So to give 180 cGy with a dose rate of 0.748 cGy/MU:

$$\text{MU} = \frac{180 \text{ cGy}}{0.748 \frac{\text{cGy}}{\text{MU}}} \approx 241 \text{ MU}$$

Answer 6

S_c is a measure of the collimator scatter and S_p is a measure of the phantom (tissue) scatter. Remember that photons interacting in the head of the machine tend to scatter (from the target, flattening filter, jaws, etc.) and enter the patient at various angles (S_c). Once the photons enter the patient, they are scattered again (S_p). S_c and S_p are therefore functions of the field size primarily since more scatter occurs at larger field apertures. Since they are correction factors they are typically close to 1 but may range from 0.9 for small fields to 1.1 for large fields. Sometimes for simplicity they are combined into a single term, $S_{c,p}$ which is simply $S_c \times S_p$. Note that the field size for S_c is defined at the isocenter. However, the field size for S_p is defined at depth, since the internal scatter can change as the beam diverges with depth.

Gibbons J, Antolak JA, Followill DS, et al. Monitor unit calculations for external photon and electron beams: Report of the AAPM Therapy Physics Committee Task Group No. 71. *Med Phys*. 2014;41(3):031501.

Question 7
How is the collimator scatter factor S_c measured?

Question 8
How is the phantom scatter factor S_p measured?

Question 9
Now suppose that a 6 MV beam is again unconventionally calibrated to deliver 1.5 cGy/MU to d_{max} (1.5 cm) at a source to skin distance of 100 cm via a 10 cm × 10 cm field in water. The percent depth dose (PDD) at 10 cm for a 6 MV beam is roughly 66%. How many monitor units (MUs) would be necessary to deliver 100 cGy to 10 cm via a 5 cm × 5 cm field in water? Assume S_c = 0.967 and S_p = 0.974.

Question 10
Now the 6 MV beam is calibrated as per the usual convention [1 cGy/MU (monitor unit) at d_{max} with a field size of 10 cm × 10 cm at the surface at a source to skin distance (SSD) of 100 cm]. Calculate the cGy/MU delivered at 10 cm via a 5 cm × 5 cm field with an extended SSD of 110 cm. Assume the percent depth dose (10 cm) continues to be 66%, S_c is 0.951 and S_p is 0.954.

Answer 7

S_c is the ratio of output for a given field size to a reference field size (10 cm × 10 cm) in air measured at isocenter (100 cm). It can be measured with an ion chamber with a build-up cap.

Answer 8

S_p is the ratio of dose for a given field size to a reference field size (10 cm × 10 cm) in a phantom at d_{max} with identical collimator opening. Theoretically it could be measured using phantoms of various sizes with a larger collimator opening. But in practice it is measured indirectly using the following equation:

$$S_p = S_{c,p} / S_c$$

where $S_{c,p}$ is the total scatter factor and defined as the ratio of dose for a given field size to reference field size (10 cm × 10 cm) in phantom at depth of maximum dose (d_{max}). $S_{c,p}$ is defined at d_{max} but actual measurements are done at larger depths (ie, 10 cm) to avoid electron contamination and converted to d_{max} using tabulated PDD values.

Answer 9

This is the same as question 3 but with a smaller field size. In Question 3, S_c and S_p were essentially counted as 1 because the field size was constant between the calibration conditions and the conditions we were interested in. Now that the field size changed, we need to introduce S_c and S_p in the equation:

$$MU = \frac{D}{D_0' \times S_c \times S_p \times PDD}$$

$$MU = \frac{100 \text{ cGy}}{\left(1.5 \dfrac{cGy}{MU}\right) \times 0.967 \times 0.974 \times 0.66} = 107.3 \approx 107$$

Note that the number of MUs required is slightly higher than before due to a smaller field size. This is due to "increased scatter" as represented by S_c and S_p.

Answer 10

This question requires both an inverse-square correction and a correction for $S_{c,p}$:

$$\frac{Dose}{MU} \text{ at depth} = \left(\frac{Dose}{MU} \text{ at reference}\right) \times PDD \times S_c \times S_p \times \left(\frac{SSD_0 + d_{max}}{SSD + d_{max}}\right)^2$$

$$\frac{Dose}{MU} \text{ at depth} = \left(1 \frac{cGy}{MU}\right) \times 0.66 \times 0.951 \times 0.954 \times \left(\frac{100 + 1.5 \text{ cm}}{110 + 1.5 \text{ cm}}\right)^2$$

$$\frac{Dose}{MU} \text{ at depth} = 0.496 \frac{cGy}{MU}$$

Question 11

In the AAPM TG-71 report, what is the equation used to perform a monitor unit (MU) calculation using source to skin distance (SSD) technique?

Question 12

A patient is treated with 6 MV photons to 100 cGy via a 10 cm × 10 cm field to 8 cm depth at 100 cm source to skin distance (SSD). The percent depth dose (PDD) at this point is 74.3%.

How many monitor units (MU) are required? Assume the calibration conditions of 1 cGy/MU to d_{max} (1.5 cm) with a 10 cm × 10 cm field size.

Question 13

The source to skin distance (SSD) changes to 115 cm. How many monitor units (MUs) are now required? Use the percent depth dose (PDD) method. Field size is kept at 10 cm × 10 cm at SSD. S_c (8.7 cm) = 0.995.

Answer 11

So far we have answered these questions using "dose rate" notation but this is not the same format used by the official reports. With a bit of algebra you will see that the two methods are equivalent. The following equation is a simple form of the MU calculation formula and a great starting place for understanding MU calculations. Note that this simplified equation does not account for off-axis point calculations, wedges, or blocks which will be covered in the next questions:

$$MU = \frac{D}{D_0' \times S_c(r_c) \times S_p(r_{d_0}) \times PDD_N(d, r, SSD) \times \left(\frac{SSD_0 + d_0}{SSD + d_0}\right)^2}$$

D: The dose at the point of interest.

D_0': Dose per MU under calibration conditions.

d: Depth of the point of calculation.

d_0: The normalization depth for photon and electron dosimetry, typically d_{max}.

r_c: The side of the equivalent square for the collimator field size defined at isocenter.

r_d: The side of the equivalent square for the field size incident on the patient, defined at the surface and at depth d, respectively.

S_c: Collimator scatter factor.

S_p: Phantom scatter factor.

Gibbons J, Antolak JA, Followill DS, et al. Monitor unit calculations for external photon and electron beams: Report of the AAPM Therapy Physics Committee Task Group No. 71. *Med Phys.* 2014;41(3):031501.

Answer 12

Remember that at calibration conditions (10 cm × 10 cm, SSD = 100 cm), $S_{c,p} = 1$. Therefore,

$$MU = \frac{D}{D_0' \cdot S_c(r_c) \times S_p(r_{d_0}) \times PDD_N(d, r, SSD) \times \left(\frac{SSD_0 + d_0}{SSD + d_0}\right)^2}$$

$$MU = \frac{100 \text{ cGy}}{1 \frac{cGy}{MU} \times 0.743 \times \left(\frac{100 \text{ cm} + 1.5 \text{ cm}}{100 \text{ cm} + 1.5 \text{ cm}}\right)^2} = 134.6 \text{ MU} \approx 135 \text{ MU}$$

Answer 13

Since the SSD has now changed, we must first convert the PDD using the Mayneord factor:

$$F = \left(\frac{SSD_1 + d}{SSD_2 + d} \times \frac{SSD_2 + D_{max}}{SSD_1 + D_{max}}\right)^2$$

$$F = \left(\frac{100 \text{ cm} + 8 \text{ cm}}{115 \text{ cm} + 8 \text{ cm}} \times \frac{115 \text{ cm} + 1.5 \text{ cm}}{100 \text{ cm} + 1.5 \text{ cm}}\right)^2 = 1.0157$$

So $PDD_2 = 0.743 \times 1.0157 = 0.755$

$$r_c = \frac{100}{115} 10 \approx 8.7 \text{ cm}$$

$$MU = \frac{D}{D_0' \cdot S_c(r_c) \times S_p(r_{d_0}) \times PDD_2(d, r, SSD) \times \left(\frac{SSD_0 + d_0}{SSD + d_0}\right)^2}$$

$$MU = \frac{100 \text{ cGy}}{1 \frac{cGy}{MU} \times 0.995 \times 0.755 \left(\frac{100 \text{ cm} + 1.5 \text{ cm}}{115 \text{ cm} + 1.5 \text{ cm}}\right)^2} = 175.4 \text{ MU}$$

Question 14

Solve the previous question (Question 13) using the tissue maximum ratio (TMR) method. TMR $(d = 8 \text{ cm}, r = 10 \text{ cm}) = 0.830$, TMR $(d = 8 \text{ cm}, r = 11 \text{ cm}) = 0.837 \, S_p (11 \text{ cm}) = 1.003$

$$r_{d = 8 \text{ cm}} = \frac{123}{115} 10 = 10.7 \text{ cm}$$

Question 15

Write the equation TG-71 uses for monitor unit (MU) calculation of beams designed with source to axis distance (SAD) technique. This time, account for blocks, wedges, and off-axis calculations.

Question 16

124 monitor units (MUs) are required to deliver a single 1 Gy fraction to a target. 50% of the field size is then blocked to save normal tissue. $S_{c,p}$ drops from 1 to 0.889 and the tissue maximum ratio (TMR) decreases from 0.782 to 0.747. How many MUs are now necessary to deliver the same dose to the target?

Answer 14

$$S_p(r_d) \approx 1.002, \text{TMR } (8, 10.7) \sim 0.835$$

$$MU = \frac{D}{D_0' \cdot S_c(r_c) \times S_p(r_d) \times \text{TMR}(d, r_d) \times \left(\dfrac{SSD_0 + d_0}{SPD}\right)^2}$$

$$MU = \frac{100 \text{ cGy}}{1\dfrac{\text{cGy}}{\text{MU}} \times 0.995 \times 1.003 \times 0.835 \times \left(\dfrac{100 \text{ cm} + 1.5 \text{ cm}}{115 \text{ cm} + 8 \text{ cm}}\right)^2} \approx 176 \text{ MU}$$

This shows the level of equivalence between calculating with TMR or percent depth dose (PDD).

Answer 15

For SAD technique, the equation in Question 11 changes to adjust for the SAD technique. Rather than the $SSD + d_0$, the source-point distance is used. Rather than percent depth dose, the tissue phantom ratio (TPR) is substituted:

$$MU = \frac{D}{D_0' \times S_c(r_c) \times S_p(r_d) \times \text{TPR}(d, r_d) \times \text{WF}(d, r_d, x) \times \text{TF} \times \text{OAR}(d, x) \times \left(\dfrac{SSD_0 + d_0}{SPD}\right)^2}$$

Source-point distance (SPD): The distance from the X-ray physical source to the plane perpendicular to the central axis that contains the point of calculation (also called SAD for source to axis distance).

$\text{TPR}(d, r_d)$ Tissue phantom ratio: The ratio of the dose rate at a given depth in phantom to the dose rate at the normalization depth for a given field size.

$\text{OAR}(d, x)$: Off-axis ratio, accounts for the nonflat profile of the beam.

$\text{WF}(d, r_d, x)$: Wedge factor, accounts for the change in output with a wedge.

Answer 16

Blocking reduces scatter and will increase the MUs necessary to deliver dose to a target. Notice that the TMR decreases with a smaller field size. Finally, most factors in the MU equation cancel out and only the $S_{c,p}$ and TMR are necessary to answer this question:

$$MU = \frac{D \times 100}{D_0' \times S_c(r_c) \times S_p(r_d) \times \text{TMR}(d, r_d) \times \left(\dfrac{SSD_0 + d_0}{SPD}\right)^2}$$

$$\frac{MU2}{MU1} = \frac{\dfrac{D \times 100}{D_0' \times 0.889 \times 0.747\left(\dfrac{SSD_0 + d_0}{SPD}\right)^2}}{\dfrac{D \times 100}{D_0' \times 1 \times 0.782\left(\dfrac{SSD_0 + d_0}{SPD}\right)^2}}$$

$$\frac{MU2}{MU1} = \frac{1 \times 0.782}{0.889 \times 0.747} = 1.18$$

$$MU2 = 124 \times 1.18 = 146$$

Question 17

A physician wants to treat a lesion at 10 cm depth with 6 MV photons using a 10 cm × 10 cm square field. The prescription is to deliver 180 cGy to the 90% isodose line. Calculate the monitor unit (MU) required for a source to skin distance (SSD) = 100 cm setup (calibration: 1 cGy/MU at d_{max}, SSD 100 cm, 10 cm × 10 cm field at SSD).

Question 18

Consider the following anterior to posterior (AP) treatment setup for a heterogeneous medium ($d_1 = d_2 = d_3 = 5$ cm). The beam's eye view of the 16 cm × 12 cm 6 MV field is shown with part of the beam blocked. The linear accelerator (linac) is calibrated to deliver 1 MU/cGy at 1.5 cm depth with source to skin distance (SSD) of 100 cm. Find the total monitor units (MUs) required to deliver 2 Gy at point P that is located at beam isocenter if electron density of the medium in the middle is same as water.

Field Size	S_c	S_p	TMR					
			$d = 11$ cm	$d = 12$ cm	$d = 14$ cm	$d = 15$ cm	$d = 16$ cm	$d = 17$ cm
16 × 16	1.009	1.018	0.786	0.761	0.711	0.688	0.665	0.641
14 × 14	1.006	1.012	0.779	0.754	0.729	0.680	0.656	0.632
12 × 12	1.003	1.006	0.770	0.744	0.693	0.667	0.643	0.619

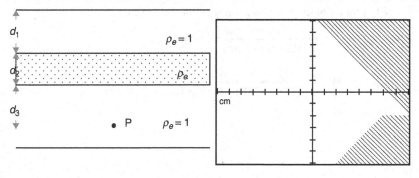

Question 19

Repeat previous question (Question 18), assuming the electron density of the medium in the middle is 1.25 relative to water.

Answer 17

Percent depth dose (PDD) for 6 MV photons at 10 cm depth is 67%. We want to deliver $180/0.90 = 200$ cGy to central axis. From the definition of PDD,

$$200 = \frac{D_{max} \times 67}{100}$$

$$D_{max} = 298.5 \text{ cGy}$$

Since the linac is calibrated to deliver 1 cGy/MU at d_{max} for 10 cm $\times$ 10 cm field at SSD of 100 cm, we need 298.5 MU.

Answer 18

$$MU = \frac{D}{D'_0 \times S_c(r_c) \times S_p(r_d) \times TMR(d, r_d) \times \left(\dfrac{SSD_0 + d_0}{SPD}\right)^2}$$

$$\left(\frac{SSD_0 + d_0}{SPD}\right)^2 = 1.03$$

From the beam's eye view, 25% of the field is blocked. So total area unblocked is $16 \times 12 \times 0.75 = 144$ cm^2.

Equivalent square (r_d) for the blocked field is roughly $\sqrt{144 \text{ cm}^2} = 12$ cm.

Equivalent square (r_c) for S_c is $\dfrac{4 \times 16 \text{ cm} \times 12 \text{ cm}}{2 \times (12 \text{ cm} + 16 \text{ cm})} \approx 14$ cm

$$MU = \frac{200 \text{ cGy}}{1 \times 1.006 \times 1.006 \times 0.667 \times 1.03} \approx 288$$

Answer 19

Equivalent depth, $d_{eq} = d_1 + \rho_e d_2 + d_3 = 5 + 1.25 \times 5 + 5 = 16.25$ cm

Use interpolation for TMR $(16.25 \text{ cm}, 12 \times 12) = 0.619 + 0.25(0.643 - 0.619) = 0.625$:

$$MU = \frac{D}{D'_0 \times S_c(r_c) \times S_p(r_d) \times TMR(d, r_d) \times ((SSD_0 + d_0)/SPD)^2 \times CF}$$

Correction Factor, $CF = \dfrac{TMR(16.25 \text{ cm}, 12 \times 12 \text{ cm})}{TMR(15 \text{ cm}, 12 \times 12 \text{ cm})} = \dfrac{0.625}{0.667} = 0.94$

$$MU = \frac{200 \text{ cGy}}{1 \times 1.006 \times 1.006 \times 0.667 \times 1.03 \times 0.94} \approx 306$$

160

Question 20

Repeat Question 18, assuming the electron density of the medium in the middle is 0.25 relative to water.

Question 21

By approximately how much does the dose rate of cobalt-60 (Co-60) decrease in one month?

Question 22

Which has a larger geometric penumbra—a cobalt-60 (Co-60) machine or a modern linear accelerator?

Question 23

To calibrate a linear accelerator we use an ion chamber to relate the output of the machine as measured by monitor units to the dose delivered under certain conditions. Explain how a cobalt-60 machine is calibrated.

Answer 20

Equivalent depth, $d_{eq} = d_1 + \rho_e d_2 + d_3 = 5 + 0.25 \times 5 + 5 = 11.25$ cm

Interpolation of TMR $(11.25$ cm, $12 \times 12) = 0.744 + 0.25(0.770 - 0.744) = 0.751$

Correction Factor, $CF = \dfrac{\text{TMR}(11.25 \text{ cm}, 12 \times 12 \text{ cm})}{\text{TMR}(15 \text{ cm}, 12 \times 12 \text{ cm})} = \dfrac{0.751}{0.667} = 1.13$

$$MU = \frac{200 \text{ cGy}}{1 \times 1.006 \times 1.006 \times 0.667 \times 1.03 \times 1.13} \approx 255$$

Answer 21

A "rule of thumb" is that cobalt decays by approximately 1% per month. While this is a good answer to remember for estimation, it will not work over a long period of time. The precise answer, using the 5.26 year half-life is $e^{-0.693 \times 1 \text{ month}/(12 \text{ months/year} \times 5.26 \text{ years})} = 1.09\%$.

Answer 22

Typically Co-60 machines have a larger geometric penumbra because the cobalt source usually is a cylinder roughly 1 to 2 cm in diameter as opposed to the roughly 3 mm diameter pencil beam of electrons that interacts with a Tungsten target in the linear accelerator (linac) head.

Answer 23

Cobalt-60 machines are controlled using a timer. Because the source is always "on," it is held inside the shielded head of the machine. When the patient is in position, the shield is removed. Calibration, therefore, is performed by measuring the time it takes for the source to deposit dose, which is a function of the activity of the source. A fresh source typically has a dose rate of 240 cGy/min at a source to axis distance (SAD) of 80 cm.

Question 24

A single-fraction dose requires 5 min to deliver on a cobalt-60 machine without accounting for a 26-s time correction. What is the total time required to deliver the fraction?

Question 25

A dose of 250 cGy is prescribed to a depth of 5 cm. The patient is treated at 100 cm source to skin distance using a 6 MV with a field size of 16 cm × 12 cm. How many monitor units (MUs) should be delivered?

$S_{c,p} = 1.023$, PDD (5, 13.7, 100) = 0.877

Question 26

A 36 cm long field is necessary to treat the entire spinal column of a patient. The spinal column is at an average depth of 5.0 cm. The patient is treated at an extended source to skin distance of 115 cm of 6 MV. The collimator jaw is set to 30 cm × 4 cm. Use the tissue maximum ratio (TMR) method to calculate the required monitor unit (MU) if the prescription dose is 300 cGy. Use S_c (7.1) = 0.987, S_p (8.5) = 0.996 and TMR (5, 8.5) = 0.921.

Question 27

A 36 cm long field is necessary to treat the entire spinal column of a patient. The spinal column is at an average of 5.0 cm depth. The patient is treated at an extended source to skin distance (SSD) of 115 cm of 6 MV. The collimator jaw is set to 30 cm × 4 cm. Use the percent depth dose (PDD) method to calculate the required monitor unit (MU) if the prescription dose is 300 cGy. Use PDD (5, 7.096, 100) = 0.858, S_c (7.1) = 0.987 and S_p (8.1) = 0.995.

Answer 24

The time correction accounts for the time it takes to move the shielding away from the cobalt source. For a fraction of this time, the source is not entirely exposed and is not delivering the full dose rate. Therefore, the time error is added onto the time it takes to deliver the source. The final time it takes to deliver this fraction is simply 5 min and 26 s.

Answer 25

Equivalent square: 4 (anterior/posterior [A/P]) = $4 \times 3.4 = 13.7$ cm

Look up data tables from a specific machine to find:

MU = $250/(0.877 \times 1.023) = 278.7 = 279$

$S_{c,p} = 1.023$, PDD (5, 13.7, 100) = 0.877

Answer 26

Equivalent square: 4 (anterior/posterior [A/P]) = 7.06 cm

Projected equivalent square size at the treatment depth = 8.5 cm

TMR (5, 8.5) = 0.921

S_c (7.1) S_p (8.5) = $0.987 \times 0.996 = 0.983$

SAD factor = $(101.5/(SSD + d))^2 = 0.715$

MU = $300/(0.983 \times 0.921 \times 0.715) = 464$

Answer 27

Equivalent field size: 4 (anterior/posterior [A/P]) = 7.06

Projected equivalent field size at 115 cm SSD = 8.1 cm

PDD (5, 7.06, 100) = 0.858

F factor = $((115 + 1.5)/(115 + 5))^2/((100 + 5)/(100 + 1.5))^2 = 0.942 \times 1.07 = 1.008$

PDD (5, 8.1, 115) = 0.864

S_c (7.1) S_p (8.1) = $0.987 \times 0.995 = 0.982$

SSD factor = $(101.5/(115 + 1.5))^2 = 0.759$

MU = $300/(0.982 \times 0.864 \times 0.759) = 464$

6

BASIC TREATMENT PLANNING

JEFF KITTEL, LISA ZICKEFOOSE, AND DIANA MATTSON

Question 1

Why is a 5° posteriorly tilted gantry angle necessary in whole brain treatment?

Question 2

What is the main advantage of treating patients in the prone position with a belly board for patients with rectal cancer?

Question 3

What is bolus?

Question 4

What is the definition of a hot spot in an external beam plan?

Answer 1

With a patient in supine position, a 5° posteriorly tilted gantry angle resulting in 275° gantry angle from the patient's right and 85° gantry angle from the patient's left, will avoid the divergence of the beams into the lenses and minimize the lens dose.

Answer 2

A belly board has an indented space for the entire abdomen to fall into, displacing the small bowel more anteriorly and further separating it from the tumor target volume, and minimizing the radiation dose to the small bowel. Another frequently used technique that also decreases the amount of small bowel in the field is to treat the patient with a full bladder. The full bladder will push the tumor volume inferiorly and separate the small bowel away from the tumor volume.

Answer 3

Bolus is any material (typically water equivalent) added on or near the patient surface. The use of bolus is to increase the surface (skin) dose when the tumor volume is located superficially. Sometimes bolus is also used to compensate for missing tissue such as in the treatment of an orbit when the eye has been removed.

Answer 4

A hot spot is a small volume that receives the highest radiation dose, higher than the prescribed dose of the target volume. In conventional radiation therapy, prior to the use of three-dimensional (3D) images and dose calculation, a hot spot was defined as an area encompassing 2 cm^2 contiguous area that receives the highest radiation dose. In 3D conformal therapy (3DCRT), a hot spot is defined as a volume (0.03 mL) receiving the highest radiation dose.

Question 5

When parallel opposed fields (anterior-posterior and posterior-anterior [AP/PA]) are used to treat a tumor in the chest region and the isocenter is located at mid-depth, in which field is the length of cord treated longer?

Question 6

What is the geometric penumbra (P) at the skin given the following data: source size = 2 cm, source to skin distance (SSD) = 100 cm, source to collimator distance (SCD) = 56 cm?

Question 7

What happens to the size of the penumbra at a depth of 10 cm? (Assume the other parameters from Question 6 remain the same.)

Question 8

What would be the equivalent square for an open 8 cm × 24 cm field size?

Answer 5

The cord is located posteriorly in the patient body. Therefore, the length of cord included in the anterior field is greater than that in the posterior field due to beam divergence. The two beams treat the same area only at the depth of the isocenter.

Answer 6

Use the following formula:

$$P = \text{source size} \times \frac{\text{SSD} + \text{depth} - \text{SCD}}{\text{SCD}}$$

$$P = 2 \times \frac{100 - 56}{56}$$

$$P = 1.57 \text{ cm.}$$

Answer 7

$$P = 2 \times \frac{100 + 10 - 56}{56}$$

$$P = 1.93 \text{ cm}$$

Penumbra (P) width increases with an increase in depth assuming source to skin distance (SSD), source to collimator distance (SCD), and source size remain the same.

Answer 8

Use the following formula:

$$EQ = 4 \times \frac{a}{p}$$

$$EQ = 4 \times \frac{(8 \times 24)}{(8 + 8 + 24 + 24)}$$

$$EQ = 12 \text{ cm}$$

Where a is the area and p is the perimeter. The equivalent square has the same percent depth dose (PDD) as the rectangle, and can be used for monitor unit calculation for the rectangle. The formula is based on equating the ratio of area/perimeter between the square and rectangle.

Question 9

A 20 cm × 20 cm field size at 100 cm source to skin distance (SSD) will be projected to what size at a depth of 15 cm from the skin?

Question 10

What is the principal advantage of isocentric techniques over source to skin distance (SSD) technique for a treatment with multiple fields?

Question 11

What is the wedge transmission factor if the output without the wedge is 222 cGy/MU and the output with the wedge at the same point is 125 cGy/MU?

Question 12

An object that measures 4 cm is placed on the patient's skin at 100 cm source to skin distance (SSD). Its image on the radiograph measures 5.4 cm. What is the target to film distance (TFD)?

Answer 9

The field size at a depth of 15 cm will be projected to 23 cm × 23 cm using the following similar triangles formula:

$$\frac{\text{Field size @ SSD1}}{\text{Field size @ SSD2}} = \frac{\text{SSD1}}{\text{SSD2}}$$

$$\frac{20}{X} = \frac{100}{115}$$

$$X = 23.$$

Answer 10

The isocentric technique eliminates the need to move the patient between fields. The isocenter is placed within the patient at a planned depth and the beams are directed from different directions. This technique relies primarily on the accuracy of machine isocentricity and not on the skin marks which can be unreliable points of reference.

Answer 11

The wedge transmission factor is 0.563 using the following formula:

$$\frac{125\,\text{cGy/MU}}{222\,\text{cGy/MU}} = 0.563$$

The wedge transmission factor (or simply *wedge factor*) is defined as the ratio of output with the wedge divided by the output without the wedge. Due to the large thickness of the wedge, the wedge factor makes a substantial adjustment in monitor units.

Answer 12

The TFD is 135 cm using the following formula:

$$\text{TFD} = \frac{\text{TOD} \times \text{image size}}{\text{object size}}$$

$$\text{TFD} = \frac{100 \times 5.4}{4}$$

where TOD is the target object distance. As the object is on the skin, the TOD equals the SSD.

Question 13

What is the main advantage for treating patients with breast cancer in a prone position?

Question 14

When planning for whole breast treatment using tangent fields, how is the separation defined? At what separation should one consider increasing the beam energy from 6 to 10 MV to maintain a uniform dose distribution?

Question 15

Calculate the field gap on the patient's skin surface for the following two fields to be matched at a depth of 5 cm from the skin surface.

12 cm $W \times 20$ cm L at 100 cm source to skin distance (SSD)
12 cm $W \times 24$ cm L at 100 cm SSD

Question 16

Calculate the angle of the lateral tangent beam for a breast treatment if the medial tangent beam is at the gantry angle of 56° and a symmetric field size of 10 cm (Width) and 18 cm (Length) at 100 cm source to axis distance (SAD) is used.

Answer 13

For patients with the tumor cavity away from the chest wall or for patients with pendulous breasts, treating these patients in a prone position decreases the radiation dose to the lungs and heart. Another method to reduce radiation dose to the heart for patients with left-sided breast cancer is to treat patient with a breath-hold technique.

Answer 14

The separation is measured as the distance between the entrances of two tangential beams. If the separation exceeded 23 cm, increasing the beam energy from 6 to 10 MV can improve dose uniformity inside the breast (<110% of the prescription dose).

Answer 15

The gap would be 1.1 cm on the skin surface for these fields using the following formula:

$$\left(\frac{L_1}{2} \times \frac{d}{SSD}\right) + \left(\frac{L_2}{2} \times \frac{d}{SSD}\right)$$

where L_1 is the length of the first field, L_2 is the length of the second field, and d is the depth at which the fields are to be matched

$$\left(\frac{20}{2} \times \frac{5}{100}\right) + \left(\frac{24}{2} \times \frac{5}{100}\right) = 1.1 \text{ cm.}$$

Answer 16

According to the formula, $\tan^{-1}\left(\frac{1}{2}W / SAD\right) = \text{Divergence}$

Opposed tangent angle = Angle + 180° − (2 × divergence)

$$\tan^{-1}\left(\frac{1}{2} \times \frac{10}{100}\right) = 2.86$$

$$56° + 180° - (2 \times 2.86) = 230.28°.$$

Question 17
A physician wants to treat a patient with medulloblastoma using four craniospinal fields (two lateral brain fields and two spinal fields). The brain field is 20 cm long with a source to skin distance (SSD) of 100 cm and designed using a half beam block technique. The spinal fields are 40 and 20 cm with a skin gap between them. Both spinal fields are designed at SSD of 100 cm. The junction point is at depth of 7 cm. Where do the hot and cold spots happen?

Question 18
What can be done to avoid or minimize the effects of cold and hot spots?

Question 19
What is the dose from each field at the junction point?

Question 20
Draw a diagram and calculate the skin gap for the spinal fields.

Answer 17

The cold spots happen between the gap left on the skin surface and junction point. The hot spot occurs where the beams overlap at depth.

Answer 18

A procedure called "feathering" is usually performed by changing the position of field edges between fractions during the course of the treatment. This way hot and cold spots are moved around and their effects are diffused.

Answer 19

The dose from each field is 50% of the prescribed dose at the same depth for each field. This way a uniform dose is achieved throughout the treatment area at the same depth.

Answer 20

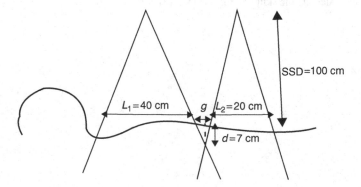

Using similar triangles formed by the two fields:

$$g = \frac{L_1}{2} \times \frac{d}{\text{SSD}} + \frac{L_2}{2} \times \frac{d}{\text{SSD}} = 20 \times 0.07 + 10 \times 0.07 = 2.1 \text{ cm.}$$

Question 21
The physician decides to treat a smaller area to avoid field matching. He would like to treat with one spinal field using an extended source to skin distance (SSD) technique because of field size limitation (maximum 40 cm × 40 cm). What should the new SSD be to treat an area of 50 cm at the skin surface?

Question 22
What is the procedure to match the spinal and cranial fields?

Question 23
How much collimator rotation is necessary to match a cranial field to the upper spine field of Question 20?

Answer 21

$$SSD = \frac{50}{40} \times 100 = 125 \text{ cm}.$$

Answer 22

If the cranial field is nondivergent (half-beam block technique used) then collimator rotation alone is sufficient to provide geometric match between the two fields. If the cranial beams are diverging, then a couch kick toward the gantry is also necessary.

Answer 23

A beam's eye view of the cranial field and a lateral view of the spinal field are shown in the figure. The collimator angle is found by calculating the diverging angle of the spinal field:

$$\tan\theta = \frac{L_1/2}{SSD}$$

$$\theta = \tan^{-1}\left(\frac{L_1}{2SSD}\right) = \tan^{-1}\left(\frac{20}{100}\right) = 11.5°$$

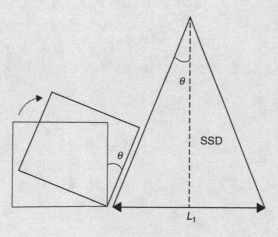

Question 24

Assume that the cranial field measures 20 cm × 20 cm and is also diverging (not half beam blocked). The source to axis distance (SAD) is 100 cm. Find the couch angle necessary to match the two orthogonal field borders.

Question 25

If a linear accelerator has an output of 1 cGy/MU at 100 cm source to skin distance (SSD) what would the output be at 120 cm SSD?

Question 26

By approximately how much does the dose increase behind 5 cm of healthy lung tissue in the path of a 10 MV photon beam?

Answer 24

The angle of the couch kick is the angle of divergence of the cranial field, found by the formula $\tan^{-1}(1/2 \text{ Field Size/SAD}) = \tan^{-1}(10 \text{ cm}/100 \text{ cm}) = 5.7°$.

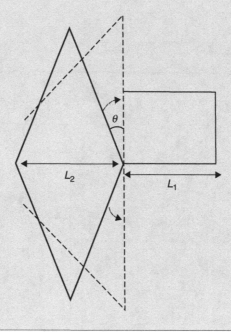

Answer 25

Use the inverse square law:

$$\text{Output at new SSD} = (\text{old SSD/new SSD})^2 \times \text{output at old SSD}$$

$$= (100/120)^2 \times 1 \text{ cGy/MU}$$

$$= 0.694 \text{ cGy/MU}.$$

Answer 26

Approximately 10%. There is an increase in dose beyond healthy lung tissue by approximately 2% per cm of lung for a 10 MV photon beam.

Question 27

When treating a patient for breast cancer, what would decrease the scatter dose to the contralateral breast?

Question 28

When using tangent fields to treat the breast and intra-mammary (IM) nodes, the medial field edge is set 3 cm to the contralateral side and the lateral field edge is set to encompass all of the breast tissue. If these fields result in inclusion of too much lung, what can be done to decrease the lung dose?

Question 29

A 24 cm × 20 cm field size is used to treat a patient's pelvis at 100 cm source to axis distance (SAD) with parallel opposed fields to the midplane. The patient's separation is 20 cm. Calculate the field size on the patient's skin.

Question 30

A physician wishes to treat a posterior spine with a field size of 10 cm × 50 cm on a linear accelerator with a maximum collimator opening of 40 cm × 40 cm at 100 cm source to skin distance (SSD). What is the minimum SSD that can be set to achieve the 10 × 50 field size?

Answer 27

To decrease the scatter dose to the contralateral breast, physical wedges on the medial tangent should be avoided.

Answer 28

The lung dose can be reduced by using a separate IM electron field that is matched with the tangents instead of using the wide tangent technique described earlier.

Answer 29

21.6 cm $\times$ 18 cm
This can be solved by similar triangles.
$24/100 = x/90$ $20/100 = y/90$.

Answer 30

This can be solved by setting up a direct proportion
$40/100 = 50/$required SSD
Required SSD $= 125$ cm.

Question 31

The dose rate in air is 111 cGy/min at 80 cm source to axis distance (SAD). The dose rate in tissue at the same point is 76 cGy/min. What is the tissue-to-air ratio (TAR)?

Question 32

Based on International Commission on Radiation Units and Measurement (ICRU) target volume definitions, identify all target definitions in increasing volume order.

Question 33

What are the definitions of "treated volume" and "irradiated volume"?

Question 34

Per the International Commission on Radiation Units and Measurement (ICRU), what accuracy is necessary when delivering dose?

Answer 31

TAR is the ratio of the dose in tissue to the dose in air at the same point. Therefore, 76 cGy/min/111 cGy/min = 0.685.

Answer 32

Gross tumor volume (GTV) < clinical target volume (CTV) < integrated target volume (ITV) < planning target volume (PTV). GTV is the visible tumor on imaging and the physical examination. The CTV is regions with concern for subclinical (microscopic) spread. The ITV adjusts for known motion in the tumor (eg, breathing). The PTV adjusts for random setup error.

Answer 33

Treated volume is the volume enclosed by the prescription isodose line. Irradiated volume is the volume enclosed by 50% of the prescription isodose line.

Answer 34

The ICRU mandates that dose calculations be accurate to a level of ±5% (American Association of Physicists in Medicine Task Group-71 [AAPM TG-71]).

Question 35

According to the dose volume histogram (DVH), what is the approximate V20 of the whole lung (black dashed)?

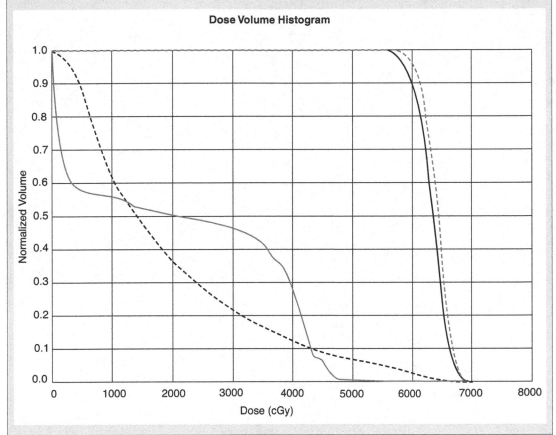

Dose Volume Histogram

Question 36

Which line likely represents the planning target volume (PTV) and the gross tumor volume (GTV)?

Question 37

What is the D90 of the planning target volume (PTV)?

Answer 35

The V20 is the volume of the organ receiving 20 Gy, which in this DVH would be approximately 38%.

Answer 36

The gray-dashed line most likely represents the GTV and the black line represents the PTV, because a small fraction of the PTV does not receive the prescription dose of 60 Gy. As the GTV is within the PTV, the GTV must receive at least as much dose as the PTV.

Answer 37

The D90 of the PTV is the dose received by 90% of the PTV. In this case, it is 60 Gy.

Question 38

How much of the whole lung receives 10 Gy or less in the dose volume histogram from Question 35? How much dose does 10% of the whole lung volume receive?

Question 39

What is the four-field box technique?

Question 40

What are the ways to match adjacent photon fields?

Question 41

What are the main dose computation algorithms used by treatment planning systems?

Answer 38

From the dose volume histogram (DVH), 61% of whole lung receives 10 Gy or less dose. 10% of the whole lung receives 44 Gy.

Answer 39

The four-field box is a treatment planning technique where four fields, spaced 90° apart, from anterior, posterior, and lateral directions form a square or rectangular shape dose distribution, similar to a box shape. This was typically used to treat prostates before intensity-modulated radiation therapy (IMRT).

Answer 40

A typical method to match adjacent photon fields is to use half beams and match them at isocenter, where there is no beam divergence. Another way is to match the divergence of the beam by angling them away from each other, as is done in cranio spinal irradiation.

Answer 41

The pencil beam, superposition convolution, and Monte Carlo algorithms. The pencil beam algorithm has been largely phased out due to its inability to accurately account for inhomogeneities, such as lung and other soft tissue.

Question 42

In 3 dimensional (3D) planning, when and how do you go "off cord"?

Question 43

When treating a spine with anterior-posterior and posterior-anterior (AP/PA) fields, how are the fields weighted?

Question 44

In a wedged pair, what direction are the wedges?

Question 45

What are the typical field borders defined for treating the whole breast with two tangent fields?

Answer 42

When treating a central target, it may be simplest to use anterior-posterior and posterior-anterior (AP/PA) fields, but this would irradiate the spinal cord as much as the target. To reduce the dose to the cord, an oblique, "off cord" field is typically added. The AP/PA fields are used to around 40 Gy, (below the cord tolerance) and then the off cord field is used.

Answer 43

Because the spine is located posteriorly, the PA field is weighted 60–70%.

Answer 44

The wedges are planned so that their heels are together. A wedged pair is used to reduce the dose where the two beams overlap the most, at the shallowest depth.

Answer 45

The typical field borders of the two tangent fields for treating the whole breast are:

Superior—1 cm above the breast tissue, which is usually just below the clavicular head.
Inferior—2 cm below the inframammary line.
Medial—The midline or midsternum.
Lateral—The midaxillary line.

Question 46
What is the density of Cerrobend relative to lead?

Question 47
What are the components of Cerrobend?

Question 48
How much does a Cerrobend block attenuate a typical beam? How many half-value layers (HVLs) of Cerrobend does this require?

Question 49
How are Cerrobend blocks shaped to minimize penumbra?

Answer 46

Approximately 83% of the density of lead.

Answer 47

50% bismuth, 26.7% lead, 13.3% tin, 10.0% cadmium.

Answer 48

Cerrobend can be sized to attenuate any amount of a beam, depending on its thickness. Typically, the block is designed to allow transmission of 5% or less. This requires n HVLs, where $(1/2)^n = 0.05$, and therefore $n = 4.3$.

Answer 49

Cerrobend blocks are "focused" toward the X-ray source by cutting them so that they match the divergence of the beam. When the blocks are cut, a Styrofoam mold is placed in a tray above a film (either a radiographic film or a digitally reconstructed radiograph [DRR]). A stylus, attached to a heated wire that anchors to a point the same distance from the Styrofoam as the source-to-block distance in the machine, is used to trace the outline of the planned block shape on the film below. The heated wire is thus angled to match the divergence of the beam originating from a source at that distance as it cuts through the Styrofoam. The cut Styrofoam is then used as a mold to pour the Cerrobend.

Question 50
What are multileaf collimators (MLCs) made from?

Question 51
How is penumbra minimized for multileaf collimators (MLCs)?

Question 52
What is the typical transmission through multileaf collimators (MLCs)?

Question 53
What are the contributions to dose under a block?

Answer 50

Tungsten.

Answer 51

Unlike cut Cerrobend blocks, MLCs are typically only focused in the direction perpendicular to the MLC movement but not focused in the direction parallel to the MLC movement (because most MLCs move in and out of the field in a straight line). The penumbra in the direction parallel to the MLC movement is thus larger than for a similarly shaped Cerrobend block. MLCs have rounded leaf edges to minimize partial transmission through the leaf edge. Blocks are also closer to the patient than MLCs, further reducing the penumbra.

Answer 52

Depending on the manufacturer, transmission through MLCs is typically approximately 2% to 4% for interleaf transmission, 1% to 2% for intraleaf transmission, and 15% to 24% between leaf ends. 2% to 4% interleaf transmission includes the use of steps or tongue in groove arrangement in between leaves.

Answer 53

There are two contributions, dose transmitted through the block, and dose scattered from outside the blocked region. The dose under the block is on the order of 10% of the unblocked dose, depending on the width of the block. A narrower block would allow more scatter under it.

Question 54
A 20-cm-thick patient is being treated with anterior-posterior parallel-opposed fields prescribed to the midplane. At what depth is the dose highest?

Question 55
If a 25-cm-thick patient is treated with anterior-posterior parallel-opposed fields prescribed to the midplane, which energy will have the smallest percentage variation between dose at the midplane and dose at D_{max}: 4 MV, 10 MV, or 16 MV?

Question 56
What is the definition of "hinge angle" for wedged fields?

Question 57
A patient has a superficial soft tissue sarcoma and the decision is made to treat using a wedged pair oriented with a hinge angle of 60°. What is the optimum wedge angle for the wedged pair?

Answer 54

At a depth of $D_{\max}$ from the anterior and posterior skin surfaces.

Answer 55

Higher energies have deeper penetration, which results in a more uniform dose distribution so 16 MV should be used.

Answer 56

The hinge angle is the angle between the central axes of the two wedged fields.

Answer 57

When two fields are angled at 60 degrees, there is a hotspot in the proximal corner. This can be reduced by adding wedges to each field. The wedges are oriented so that the heels are facing each other. The optimal wedge angle theta (θ) for any two fields oriented at angle phi (φ) is $\theta = 90 - \varphi/2$. Therefore, $\theta = 90 - 60/2 = 60°$.

Question 58

A patient is being treated with a three-field technique to the pelvis for rectal cancer. If wedges are going to be used to compensate for the differential thickness of the patient from anterior to posterior, where will the heels of the wedges be placed?

Question 59

A patient has an esophageal tumor and the decision is made to treat to 50.4 Gy. What is the downside of using unweighted anterior-posterior and posterior-anterior (AP/PA) parallel-opposed fields? What is the downside of using a four-field technique?

Question 60

As field size increases, what happens to surface dose?

Question 61

As tray-to-skin distance decreases, what happens to surface dose?

Answer 58

Wedges are applied to the lateral fields with the heels pointed posteriorly, because the patient is typically thinner toward the sacrum than the umbilicus. This also reduces hotspots from the combination of the lateral fields and the posterior field.

Answer 59

The spinal cord will get a nearly full dose or above because the hotspots will be close to the surface of the patient. Conversely, a four-field technique will result in a higher dose to the lungs.

Answer 60

It increases. There will be more electron contamination of the beam due to scatter interactions with the collimator and air.

Answer 61

It increases. Trays that are used to hold blocks are sources of electron contamination, and the closer the tray is to the surface, the less the opportunity for the electrons to scatter out of the field.

Question 62
What happens to surface dose and d_{max} when using an oblique beam?

Question 63
What is one way of increasing surface dose without decreasing penetration at depth?

Question 64
What is the difference between bolus and a compensator?

Answer 62

Surface dose increases. The maximum increase is for a tangential field, where the skin dose is approximately four times that of a perpendicular field. d_{max} decreases. It is measured perpendicularly to the skin and when the beam is oblique, it travels a longer path length to reach a particular perpendicular depth. Therefore, d_{max} occurs at a lower perpendicular depth than when the field is perpendicular to the skin.

Answer 63

Use a beam spoiler, which is a plastic tray placed in the field close to the skin surface. The beam spoiler increases electron contamination but does not significantly attenuate the beam, therefore increasing the skin dose without decreasing penetration.

Answer 64

Bolus is a uniform thickness that is intended to increase dose to the patient's skin. Compensators are intended to "compensate" for patients' variable skin contours. Compensators are specially designed for each patient. A wedge is a type of compensator that compensates in only one direction and is not customized for each particular patient.

7

ELECTRON TREATMENT

MATTHEW VOSSLER AND ANTHONY MASTROIANNI

Question 1

How do electrons lose energy in a medium?

Question 2

What is the practical range R_p for electrons?

Question 3

What effect does changing the source-to-skin distance (SSD) have on the electron depth dose curve?

Question 4

What is the field size dependence of R_{90} and R_p?

Answer 1

They lose energy through collisional interactions (ie, ionization and excitation) and radiative interactions (bremsstrahlung). In therapy, radiative losses only become significant at higher energies and high-Z materials.

Answer 2

The practical range is the depth of electron penetration. It is the point at which the tangent to the descending portion of the depth dose curve intersects with the backward extrapolation of the bremsstrahlung tail. Practical range in cm is approximately ½ E(MeV).

Answer 3

The effect is fairly minimal due to the shallowness of the penetration of the electron beam. However, for higher energies the R_{90} can be shifted distally a few mm as SSD increases.

Answer 4

When the field size is above a threshold value, there is no depth dose variation. Below this threshold (which varies with beam energy), there can be significant variation. The depth of R_{90} or range of 90% dose is shifted increasingly toward the surface as field size decreases. R_p does not change with field size as it reflects the energy of the beam only.

Question 5

How does the buildup region change with energy when using electrons?

Question 6

What are some cases where skin collimation would be preferable to using a cutout?

Question 7

What is the rough approximation for the useful depth for an electron beam as it relates to its energy?

Question 8

An electron beam will be used to treat a tumor whose most distal depth is 4.8 cm. Assume there are no critical structures beyond the tumor. What energy should be used?

Answer 5

The surface dose increases with beam energy, from approximately 75% to 95%. Skin sparing is minimal with electrons, and almost nonexistent at higher energies. This is in contrast to photons where surface dose decreases with increasing beam energy.

Answer 6

The primary benefit of skin collimation is a much sharper penumbra compared with a cutout. This is useful for:

• Small field treatments
• Providing maximal protection to adjacent critical structures
• Reducing penumbra beneath a bolus
• Reducing penumbra beneath an extended air gap
• Reducing penumbra in electron arc therapy

Answer 7

The useful depth in cm is the approximate point where the 80% to 90% isodose line occurs:
D80(cm) ~ 1/3 E(MeV) or D90(cm) ~ E(MeV)/3.3. Note that $E/4$ has also been used to approximate D90. It is important to check percent depth dose curves (PDDs) for specific field size to choose the right energy for depth of treatment required.

Answer 8

Typically, the tumor should be covered by the 90% isodose line. A rule of thumb for determining the energy to use is

$$E_{p,0} \sim 3.3 \times R_{90}(cm)$$

So in the example the energy selected would be $3.3 \times 4.8 = 15.8$, so a 16 MeV beam should be selected. To cover with the 80% isodose line, the rule of thumb is

$$E_{p,0} \sim 3 \times R_{80}(cm)$$

and so the energy would be $3 \times 4.8 = 14.4$ or 15 MeV.

Question 9

Where does the X-ray contamination of an electron beam come from, and how does it vary with energy?

Question 10

Why is bolus used in electron therapy and what kind of material is bolus made from?

Question 11

How would the depth dose for a rectangular field of width $L \times W$ be determined, if the depth doses for square fields $L \times L$ and $W \times W$ are known?

Question 12

Electron beams are ideally treated en face, or perpendicular to a flat patient surface. What is the effect of treating on a sloped, or oblique, skin surface?

Answer 9

The X-ray contamination of an electron beam results from bremsstrahlung interactions within the linac head (scattering foils, ion chambers, collimator jaws, etc.) and in patient tissues. Contamination increases with increasing energy, typical values are: 0.5% to 1% for 6 to 12 MeV, 1% to 2% for 12 to 15 MeV, and 2% to 5% for 15 to 20 MeV.

Answer 10

Bolus is used to: (1) reduce surface irregularities, (2) limit the penetration of the electron beam in certain places, and (3) increase the surface dose. Bolus is made of a tissue equivalent Z material. Commonly used bolus materials include wax, paraffin gauze, superflab, and other pliable plastics.

Answer 11

At a given depth d,

$$\%D(d, L \times W) = \sqrt{\%D(d, L \times L) \times \%D(d, W \times W)}$$

Answer 12

Treating on an oblique surface creates: increased surface dose, a higher maximum dose, a shift in R_{90} toward the surface, and an increase in R_p. These changes are most significant at angles of obliquity >30°. Beam obliquity increases side scatter at the point of maximum dose, increases the depth of penetration of the beam, and moves D_{max} deeper into the patient.

Question 13

What is the effect of treating through an air cavity? What should be done to mitigate this effect when treating through nasal passages?

Question 14

What is the effect of treating through bone?

Question 15

What is the effect of treating a protuberance (such as the nose), or a cavity (such as near the external auditory meatus)?

Question 16

What would be the effect of having 2 cm of bolus covering only part of the electron field?

Answer 13

The dose distal to the air cavity is increased. The dose lateral and distal to the air cavity is decreased (both effects are due to loss of side-scatter equilibrium). Also, the range of the electrons is increased due to lost attenuation. When treating through nasal passages (eg, the nasal septum), nose plugs should be used to replace the lost scattering medium.

Answer 14

The dose directly distal to the bone is decreased. The dose lateral and distal to the bone is increased. Again, both of these effects are due to loss of side-scatter equilibrium. With bone, there is more scatter out of the bone than into the bone. This is the opposite case to air where more radiation scatters into the air cavity than out of the cavity.

Answer 15

Surface irregularities and internal heterogeneities such as these can lead to a complex dose distribution with hot and cold spots. Typically for a protuberance the hot spots will be on either side of the protuberance, and a cold spot behind it. The base of a cavity will be hot while its sides will be cold. Bolus can help to alleviate these issues.

Answer 16

The edge of the bolus would act like a protuberance, causing a hot spot just outside the bolus and a cold spot inside the bolus. This should be avoided by tapering the edge of the bolus.

Question 17

What are the two primary considerations in designing internal collimation/shielding?

Question 18

What is the most common approach for minimizing the hot and cold spots that result from abutting electron fields?

Question 19

How is treatment planning achieved when intraoperative irradiation is performed?

Question 20

In electron arc therapy, the air gap from the secondary collimator to the patient is typically larger than normal. What issue does this cause, and how is it remedied?

Answer 17

First, the collimator must be sufficiently thick to stop the radiation. Second, backscatter from the collimator can be significant and must be taken into account by coating the shield with plastic, wax, or ceramic.

Answer 18

The degree of heterogeneity is reduced by feathering the beam edge by ±1 cm over the course of treatment.

Answer 19

Planning takes place in a surgical setting where it is not possible to CT the patient in the treatment position. Therefore manual calculations are performed, based on estimation of depth, and fields shaped using lead.

Answer 20

The large air gap causes a large penumbra. This is fixed by using skin collimation to sharpen the penumbra, and rotating the arc approximately 15° beyond the edge of the treatment area.

Question 21
What is the rule of thumb when designing the shape of the cutout aperture?

Question 22
Which of the following increase with increasing energy: surface dose, depth of D_{max}, depth of 90% isodose line, practical range, and bremsstrahlung contamination?

Question 23
Why must electron isodose curves be calculated for each machine for the same energy and field sizes?

Question 24
How does electron backscatter vary with both atomic number and energy?

Answer 21

Typically there is about a 1-cm margin between the edge of the cutout and the edge of the target volume when both are projected to isocenter.

Answer 22

All of these increase with increasing energy except for D_{max} depth, which varies irregularly with energy and machine type.

Answer 23

Scattering of electrons by different physical components in the electron beam (see Question 9).

Answer 24

Backscatter increases with increasing atomic number and decreases with increasing electron energy.

Question 25

How does one determine the dose at a point when using electron arc therapy?

Question 26

When using electron shields on a patient, what must you account for?

Question 27

What are the three significant regions in an electron depth dose distribution?

Question 28

What are the relative electron densities of compact bone, spongy bone, and lung?

Answer 25

One could measure the dose at a point in a cylindrical phantom or integrate the isodose distribution for the arc at a point.

Answer 26

The shield causes electron backscatter, which increases tissue dose proximate to the shield. As a result, it is important to cover the shield with a filter of a lower atomic number than the shield (eg, wax or plastic on eye shields).

Answer 27

(1) Buildup region caused by side-scattered electrons, which increases with electron energy, (2) regions of sharp dose falloff, beginning around the 90% isodose, and (3) the tail due to bremsstrahlung, the magnitude of the tail increases with increasing energy.

Answer 28

The relative electron densities are 1.6, 1.1, and 0.2, respectively.

Question 29

How deep will a 6 MeV beam reach into the lung if there is 1 cm of tissue, 0.5 cm of compact bone, and then 10 cm of lung?

Question 30

How do you determine the thickness of lead when making blocks to shape electron fields?

Question 31

What is the virtual source of an electron beam?

Question 32

When might you use the virtual source of an electron beam?

Answer 29

The range of a 6 MeV beam in water is 3 cm. The initial tissue is equivalent to 1 cm of water. The compact bone is 0.5 cm with a relative electron density of 1.6, therefore the effective depth in water is $0.5 \times 1.6 = 0.8$ cm of water. The beam therefore has $3 - 1 - 0.8 = 1.2$ cm of water range remaining. The range in lung is the range in water divided by the relative electron density of lung $1.2/0.2 = 6$ cm.

Answer 30

The rule of thumb is T(lead) mm = 0.5 mm/MeV. Sometimes 1 mm can be added to the thickness for safety. Cerrobend is around 20% less dense than lead, so T(Cerrobend) = $1.2 \times$ T(lead).

Answer 31

Unlike a photon beam, which has a distinct focus originating at the X-ray target, an electron beam behaves differently. It appears to originate from a virtual point in space, which can change depending on beam energy and field size. Measurements taken at different distances and plotted on a graph can be used to determine the virtual source position, which is typically just upstream of the scattering foil.

Answer 32

To calculate the virtual source to skin distance (SSD) for estimation of output at extended SSD using inverse square.

Question 33

An electron cone has an output of 1.13 cGy/MU at d_{max}. How many MU are needed to deliver 200 cGy to the 90% isodose level?

Question 34

What is the energy spectrum of an electron beam as it leaves the accelerator and reaches the patient?

Question 35

What is the energy of a 12 MeV beam at 2 cm depth in water?

Question 36

What is the difference in the isodose lines for an en face electron beam with regards to the difference between the high (90%) and low (20%) lines?

Answer 33

The basic formula for calculating MUs is:

$$MU = \frac{Dose}{Output\ factor \times Isodose\ line}$$

$$= 200/(1.13 \times 0.90)$$
$$= 197$$

Answer 34

As an electron beam leaves the accelerator, it is practically monoenergetic. On its way to the patient, it interacts with scattering foils, collimators, air, and other structures, resulting in a broadening of the energy spectrum. The mean energy at the patient's surface is lower than that of the initial beam created inside the linear accelerator.

Answer 35

$$E = E_0(1 - depth/R_p)$$

$$= 12(1 - 2/6) \qquad R_p = 12/2 \text{ (refer to Question 2)}$$

$$= 8 \text{ MeV}$$

Answer 36

For an electron beam, high isodose lines bow inward, creating a smaller region receiving the prescription isodose at depth than the field size at the surface. Conversely, the low isodose lines bow outward.

Question 37

Where is the hotspot when a 9 MeV electron beam is abutted to a 6 MV photon beam?

Question 38

What are common treatment sites for electrons?

Question 39

When are electrons used in breast irradiation?

Question 40

A physician wants to treat to 3.5 cm depth with electrons, but avoid a critical structure which is 6.5 cm deep. The available electron energies are 6, 9, 12, and 15 MeV. What energy would you use?

Question 41

When placing bolus on the skin, why must it be placed directly on the skin?

Answer 37

The isodose lines of electron beams tend to bulge outward at depth, leading to hot and cold spots. If the beams are matched at the skin, the electron beam will bulge into the photon beam at depth and create a hotspot.

Answer 38

Electrons are often used to treat superficial tumors of the skin (eyelids, nose, scalp, ear, etc.), shallow tumors, tumor beds, and scar boosts.

Answer 39

Electrons are used in the treatment of Internal Mammary Chain (IMC) nodes, chest wall post mastectomy, and tumor bed boosts.

Answer 40

To treat to the 90% isodose line, $E = 3.5 \times 3.3 = 11.55$ MeV. Electron energy of 13 MeV is required to reach a depth of 6.5 cm. Therefore a 12 MeV beam would cover the target, but not reach the critical structure.

Answer 41

Air gaps between skin and bolus will result in a decreased dose and increased penumbra as a consequence of the bolus scattering the electrons, which then can travel out of the field in the air gap.

8

BRACHYTHERAPY

MARIA RYBAK, NEIL WOODY, AND ALLAN WILKINSON

Question 1

What is brachytherapy?

Question 2

What are the types of brachytherapy?

Question 3

What are different types of brachytherapy loading systems?

Question 4

What are permanent versus temporary implants in brachytherapy?

Answer 1

Brachytherapy is a special procedure in Radiation Oncology that uses radioactive sources placed at short distances (hence *brachy*) from the target. Brachytherapy generates highly conformal dose distributions in a target volume because radioactive seeds (or sources) are placed directly within or in the vicinity of the target tissue.

Answer 2

Interstitial brachytherapy—radioactive sources are placed in the target tissue directly either permanently or temporarily.

Intracavitary brachytherapy—radioactive sources are contained in an applicator that is inserted into body cavities such as the vagina or uterus.

Intraluminal brachytherapy—subclass of intracavitary brachytherapy in which the radioactive sources are inserted in the lumen of the patient such as the blood vessel, bronchus, esophagus, or bile duct.

Surface–Radioactive sources (or seeds) are placed in the surface plaques or molds, which are then placed on the treatment area such as the eye or skin.

Answer 3

Manual "hot" loading: used for low dose rate seeds such as prostate or eye plaque.

Manual afterloading: this technique is not frequently used anymore.

Remote afterloading: most frequently used for high dose rate treatment.

Answer 4

Permanent implants—the radioactive sources are permanently implanted into the tumor, the patient is released from the hospital with radioactive materials in them.

Temporary implants—the radioactive material is implanted into or close to the tumor and is removed once the prescribed radiation dose has been delivered.

Question 5

What are the dose rate ranges for low-, medium-, and high-dose-rate brachytherapy according to International Commission for Radiation Units and Measurements (ICRU) Report No. 38?

Question 6

What radionuclides are currently most used for brachytherapy treatments?

Question 7

What types of radiation are used in brachytherapy?

Question 8

How is radiation source strength typically specified in clinic?

Answer 5

Low-Dose-Rate (LDR): 0.4 to 2.0 Gy per hour—used for permanent and manually afterloaded brachytherapy

Medium-Dose-Rate (MDR): 2 to 12 Gy per hour. Pulsed dose rate (PDR) brachytherapy afterloaders were developed in this dose rate realm to replicate the LDR experience in terms of total treatment duration but with the source exposed in pulses for only 5 to 10 minutes per hour

High-Dose-Rate (HDR): more than 12 Gy per hour—HDR brachytherapy utilizes very high activity sources, typically a 10 Ci Ir-192 source. Treatment is delivered by remote-control techniques. The usual dose rate is about 100 to 300 Gy per hour.

Answer 6

Gamma emitters: Cs-137 and Ir-192 for high energy gammas, or I-125 and Pd-103 for low energy gammas
Beta emitters: P-32, Ru-106, Sr-90, and Y-90.

Answer 7

Photons, electrons (betas), and rarely neutrons (Cf-252) and alpha particles are used.

Answer 8

For photon emitters, air kerma strength (U) is commonly used; for electron emitters, Becquerel (usually MBq or GBq) is typically used. Curie (Ci) and mCi are older units that are still commonly used for photon emitters.

Question 9

You receive an Ir-192 seed with an air kerma strength of 6.25 µGy m²/h. What is the strength of the source in mg-Ra equivalent?

Question 10

The apparent activity for the Ir-192 source is measured to be 20 mCi. Calculate the air kerma strength in cGy cm²/h (The exposure rate constant of Ir-192 is 4.69 R cm²/mCi h).

Question 11

What are the physical states of radionuclides used in brachytherapy?

Question 12

What are the advantages of the high-dose-rate (HDR) brachytherapy compared with low-dose-rate (LDR) brachytherapy?

Answer 9

1 mg-Ra equivalent is defined as 8.25×10^{-4} R/h. Using the Roentgen to rad conversion factor for air 0.876 rad/R and converting Rad (cGy) to μGy, we obtain 8.76×10^3 μGy/R.

Thus 1 mg-Ra eq at 1m = 8.25×10^{-4} R/h $\times 8.76 \times 10^3$ μGy/R = 7.23 μGy m^2/h

Dividing the air kerma strength of our source by this conversion factor gives us the result.

6.25/7.23 = 0.864 mg-Ra eq.

Answer 10

Air kerma strength = Exposure rate constant (R cm^2/mCi h) $\times$ Apparent activity (mCi) $\times$ Roentgen to cGy conversion factor for air of 0.876 cGy/R

= 4.69 R cm^2/mCi h $\times$ 20 mCi $\times$ 0.876 cGy/R

= 82.2 cGy cm^2/h

Answer 11

Solids, liquids, and gases (Xe-133). Solid sources are sealed (encapsulated in a metal shell).

Answer 12

Out-patient procedure

Safety—reduction or elimination of radiation exposure to the radiation therapy staff

Optimization—moving source allows optimization of the dose distribution by adjustment of the dwell times for each dwell position in each channel (catheter or needle), permitting very fine control of the dose distribution

Stability—HDR intracavitary treatments take less time (usually under an hour), and the movement of the applicators during treatment is minimized.

Dose reduction to normal tissue—shorter duration of HDR treatments allows for physical displacement of normal tissue structure during treatment

Applicator size—the small size of the HDR source permits the use of smaller applicators

Question 13

What are the disadvantages of the high-dose-rate (HDR) brachytherapy compared with low-dose-rate (LDR) brachytherapy?

Question 14

What are the safety features and operational interlocks of the high-dose-rate (HDR) afterloader?

Question 15

What is the current method for calculating dose rate in tissue from a radioactive source?

Question 16

What is anisotropy with respect to radioactive sources?

Answer 13

Investment—machine's cost can be anywhere between $1M and $2M.

Radiobiology—as the dose rate increases, the radiosensitivity (damage per unit dose) increases for both normal tissues and tumors, the radiosensitivity for the normal tissue increases faster, increasing the likelihood of injuring the patient while controlling the tumor. Overcoming this requires the use of the advantages of *optimization*, *geometry*, *stability*, and *dose reduction to normal tissues*, and multiple fractionation treatment.

Safety—if the HDR machine has a malfunction or if a patient has an emergency situation, the risk of accidental radiation exposure to the patient and the staff is much higher in HDR than in LDR.

Answer 14

Audio/visual system
Radiation monitors and treatment on indicator
Door interlock
Emergency shut-offs
Emergency crank
Backup battery

Answer 15

The TG-43 formalism with no heterogeneity corrections is the current standard.

Update of AAPM Task Group No. 43 Report: a revised AAPM protocol for brachytherapy dose calculations. *Med Phys*. 2004;31:633–674.

Answer 16

Anisotropy refers to the directional dependence of the fluence from a source due to the location of the radioactive material within the source and differences in wall thickness and construction.

Question 17
What is the main determinant of the dose rate from a source?

Question 18
What instrument would you use to locate a missing source?

Question 19
What instrument would you use to survey a patient before release?

Question 20
What are the requirements regarding calibration of new sources?

Answer 17

For distances greater than a few mm, it is the inverse square factor.

Answer 18

A Geiger–Muller (GM) counter.

Answer 19

A sensitive, calibrated ion chamber (eg, one with a large, pressurized gas-filled chamber) is typically used.

Answer 20

New sources must be calibrated before treating patients using a dosimetry system that has a National Institute of Standards and Technology (NIST) traceable calibration. The dosimetry system typically comprises a well-chamber and an electrometer capable of reading in the current mode. For the source activity in mCi range, the typical current readings from the electrometer are on the order of 10^{-11} A (ampere). For an HDR source (about 10 Ci activity), the current is 10^{-7} A. This current is then converted into the activity of the source.

Question 21

What are the corrections applied to the electrometer readings when performing a calibration check?

Question 22

What are the rules regarding a radioactive materials (RAM) inventory?

Question 1   **8.2 LOW-DOSE-RATE BRACHYTHERAPY**

What isotopes are used for permanent implants and what are the reasons for choosing them?

Question 2

What are the typical dosimetric parameters for a prostate implant?

Answer 21

If the well chamber is open to the atmosphere, as most are, a temperature and pressure correction must be applied. In addition, there may be an electrometer scale reading correction.

Answer 22

The Nuclear Regulatory Commission (NRC) requires a licensee to maintain an inventory log for all radioactive materials. The log must contain the type of source (isotope), source strength, and its location. Permanent sources implanted in a patient are not subject to this inventory control once the patient has been released from the facility.

Answer 1

The isotopes most commonly used are I-125, Pd-103, and Cs-131. They are used because of their low average photon energies (0.028, 0.021, and 0.029 MeV) so that they will treat only the tumor, and have relatively short half-lives (59.4, 17, and 9.7 days).

Answer 2

For I-125, the prescription dose is 144 Gy to cover the prostate delineated on the ultrasound images. V150 (volume of the prostate receiving 150% of the prescription dose of 144 Gy) values ranging from 40% to 50% of the prostate and V200 from 10% to 20% of the prostate are acceptable. Although there may be no explicit margin contoured, the implant volume receiving 144 Gy is approximately twice that of the prostate itself. For Pd-103, the prescription dose is 125 Gy.

Question 3

What are the simplifications in the TG-43 calculation used for prostate implants?

Question 4

What is the release criterion for a prostate seed implant patient?

Question 5

What is the purpose of postimplant dosimetry?

Question 6

A patient undergoes a low-dose-rate (LDR) prostate brachytherapy implant with Pd-103 to a prescription dose of 125 Gy. What is the initial dose rate (cGy/h) of the implant?

Answer 3

Per Radiation Therapy Oncology Group (RTOG) protocols, the source is modeled as a point and the anisotropy as a function of distance (r) only with no directional information about seed orientation within the implant.

Answer 4

Per Nuclear Regulatory Commission (NRC) regulations (hence also agreement states), "a licensee may authorize the release from its control of any individual who has been administered unsealed radioactive material or implants containing radioactive material if the total effective dose equivalent to any other individual from exposure to the released individual is not likely to exceed 5 millisieverts (0.5 rem)." For prostate patients, this is satisfied if the exposure rate measured at 1 m from the patient is <1 mR/h.

Answer 5

CT-based postimplant dosimetry is usually conducted roughly 30 days after a prostate seed implant procedure. This allows for gland swelling due to edema to subside. The postimplant dosimetry is primarily performed as a quality assurance measure for the implant procedure. It has also been used for regulatory purposes (ie, defining a "medical event").

Answer 6

The initial prescription dose will be equal to the total dose (125 Gy)/the average life of the source. The average life is: 1.44 times the half-life, so for Pd-103: $T_{average}$ = 17 days × 24 hours/day × 1.44 or 587.5 hours. Therefore dose rate is 125 Gy/587.5 hours = 21.3 cGy/h. By comparison, the initial dose rate for an I-125 implant of 144 Gy is about 7 cGy/h, which is lower due to its longer half-life.

Question 7

Describe a prostate seed implant procedure?

Question 8

What brachytherapy procedure is used for treating ocular lesions?

Question 9

Describe the eye plaques in current clinical use.

Question 10

How is the dose specified and calculated for eye plaque treatments?

Answer 7

The patient is placed in the dorsal lithotomy position under general anesthesia. Radioactive sources are implanted through the perineum using preloaded needles containing either loose seeds or seeds in a strand. Radioactive seeds are spaced at least 1 cm apart in the needle. The number of needles needed for an implant depends on the volume of the prostate. The needles are typically arranged to provide a modified peripheral loading, resulting in fewer sources in the center of the prostate near the urethra. The needles are inserted through a special template that is attached to a transrectal ultrasound probe. Seeds may also be implanted using a Mick applicator.

Answer 8

Uveal melanoma and retinoblastoma may be treated using a surface plaque containing radioactive material (typically I-125, Ru-106, Pd-103, or Cs-131). Melanomas are treated with a prescription dose of 85 Gy in 3 or 4 days; retinoblastomas with a prescription dose of 40 to 45 Gy in 2 days. The plaque also shields the eye cavity from radiation.

Answer 9

Collaborative Ocular Melanoma Study (COMS, begun in 1986) plaques consisting of a gold shield with a silastic insert containing the I-125 seeds as well as Eye Physics gold plaques with embedded seeds are used. There are COMS plaques available with a notch to facilitate placement near the optic nerve.

Answer 10

The Collaborative Ocular Melanoma Study (COMS) dose is 85 Gy to 5 mm or the tumor apex, whichever is greater. Treatment times are typically around 100 hours. For COMS, the dose was calculated using a point model for the seed and no anisotropy or heterogeneity correction. Current AAPM (the American Association of Physicists in Medicine) recommendations are to use a line-source approximation and calculate for homogeneous water media. Included in the Task Group (TG) report 129 are data for heterogeneous corrections. Software such as Plaque Simulator modifies the calculation by accounting for silastic carrier attenuation and changes in scatter due to the gold shield.

The American Brachytherapy Society recommendations for brachytherapy of uveal melanomas. *Int J Radiat Oncol Biol Phys*. 2003;56:544–555.

Dosimetry of 125 I and 103 Pd COMS eye plaques for intraocular tumors: report of task group 129 by the AAPM and ABS. *Med Phys*. 2012;39(10).

Question 11
What are the regulations regarding seed activity assays?

Question 12
What radiation safety precautions are taken regarding eye plaque patients?

Question 13
What radiation safety precautions are taken for prostate implant patients?

Question 14
What is the primary goal and key features of the Patterson–Parker (Manchester) system of interstitial implants?

Answer 11

The Nuclear Regulatory Commission (NRC) and hence agreement states require a 10% independent assay to confirm the accuracy of the specified seed activity. The assay may be performed by a third party, but the AAPM (the American Association of Physicists in Medicine) recommends that a check be done at the local institution.

Answer 12

Patients remain in the hospital for the duration of the therapy. The room in which they are housed requires a radiation sign posted on the outside of the room; the patients wear special leaded glasses that reduce radiation exposure levels by a factor of 5 to 6 when visitors or nursing staff are present. Nursing staff require annual radiation safety training. Following patient discharge, the room and contents are surveyed for radioactive material.

Answer 13

Following the operating room implant procedure, the patient is taken to a recovery area. He is provided with a urinal for his use. After discharge (typically a few hours), the urinal and patient bedding are checked for radioactive sources. If any sources are found, they are stored in a locked cabinet until removal by Radiation Safety. Patients with permanent implants are provided with a small card indicating the date and nature (isotope, total activity) of the implant and a document of precautions to be followed to minimize exposure to others.

Answer 14

The primary goal is to deliver a uniform dose to a plane or volume in parallel planes 0.5 cm from the implanted plane(s) (within +/− 10% of the prescribed dose). To achieve this goal, the system uses specified rules for distribution of sources and activity. For a planar implant the smaller the treated area the greater the fraction of the amount of Radium (or equivalent) to be placed at the periphery. The implant volume is determined and tables are used to determine the milligram hours of Radium per 1,000 roentgens. Note that the tables employed the historical exposure rate constant (Γ) for Radium (8.4 R cm^2/mg-h) instead of the current value for Radium $\Gamma = 8.25$ R cm^2/mg-h and thus the tables truly reflect milligram hours of Radium per 900 cGy.

Question 15

How does the Quimby system differ in their goal and source loading from the Patterson–Parker system?

Question 16

What is the goal of the Paris system and its key features?

Question 17

What sources can be employed with the Patterson–Parker and Quimby systems?

Question 18

What has largely supplanted systems such as Patterson–Parker in modern interstitial brachytherapy planning?

Answer 15

The goal of the Quimby system is to calculate the maximum dose in the center of the treatment plane at a distance of up to 3 cm. The system relies on a uniform distribution of sources of equal linear activity. By comparison the Patterson–Parker system uses nonuniform distributions and may employ varied source activities to achieve a uniform dose to a plane(s).

Answer 16

The Paris system prescribes dose to an isodose surface (reference isodose). Like the Quimby system uniform sources placed in parallel lines are employed.

Answer 17

Both systems were designed for Radium implants. Isotopes similar to Radium (Radium equivalents) Ir-192 and Cs-137 can be calculated but these systems are not compatible with lower energy brachytherapy sources such as I-125.

Answer 18

Computerized calculation of doses delivered with summation of doses to each point from all contributing sources. Furthermore use of afterloading systems allow for evaluation of the plan with dummy sources in place and active source placement after the plan has been evaluated.

Question 1

What is the most common high-dose-rate (HDR) brachytherapy source, its half-life, dimensions and typical activity?

Question 2

What is the Nuclear Regulatory Commission (NRC) limit on leakage levels for high-dose-rate (HDR) units?

Question 3

What are the steps for initiating a high-dose-rate (HDR) procedure?

Question 4

What are the advantages and disadvantages of Cs-137 as high-dose-rate (HDR) brachytherapy source relative to Ir-192?

Answer 1

Iridium-192 is the most common HDR brachytherapy source. Ir-192 has a half-life of 74.4 days and a mean energy of 380 keV. A typical source is 0.3 to 0.6 mm in diameter and 3.5 to 10 mm in length with an initial activity of ~10 Ci.

Answer 2

Leakage may not exceed 1 mR/h at a distance of 10 cm from the nearest accessible surface of the safe when the source is in the shielded position.

Answer 3

The following steps must be completed to be compliant with the Nuclear Regulatory Commission (NRC):

1. Authorized physician user must sign the complete written directive
2. Patient is identified and verified by two methods
3. Treatment plan must be checked by a medical physicist
4. Pretreatment HDR unit safety checks must be completed
5. Prior to treatment delivery the authorized user must verify patient and treatment detail
6. Treatment must be supervised from start to end by authorized user and treatment records must be recorded
7. A postdelivery survey must be completed
8. Medical events must be recorded and reported
9. Periodic reviews at least yearly are performed and source and calibration is performed and recorded

Answer 4

Cs-137 has a higher average energy than Ir-192 that could be beneficial for improved percent depth dose, but higher energies are accompanied by higher shielding requirements. Cs-137 has a longer half-life requiring less frequent replacement than Ir-192. However, Cs-137 has lower specific activity requiring a larger source and hence larger catheters.

Question 5

You have a brachytherapy source with a half-value layer (HVL) of 2 cm of lead. You are doubling the usage of this source. On one side of the high-dose-rate (HDR) suite is a bathroom and on the other side a hallway (occupancy factor ¼) that is being converted into a work area (occupancy factor 1). To maintain safe shielding levels, how many cm of lead if any should be added to the wall facing the bathroom and to the wall facing the new work area?

Question 6

Why is high-dose-rate (HDR) brachytherapy used for the treatment of endometrial cancer?

Question 7

What is the most commonly used applicator for treatment of endometrial cancer?

Question 8

In vaginal cuff brachytherapy treatment for endometrial cancer what is the preferred vaginal cylinder diameter?

Answer 5

Since the usage of the source is set to double one HVL (2 cm of lead) should be applied to all walls to maintain current shielding levels. In addition for the wall facing the new work area where the occupancy factor has increased fourfold, two additional HVL (4 cm) of shielding should be added to this wall. Therefore 2 cm on the bathroom side and 6 cm on the work area site are needed.

Answer 6

The vast majority of patients undergo curative hysterectomies, however, with no further therapy approximately 12% of the patients are likely to suffer recurrences. Patients who received prophylactic radiation to the vaginal cuff had much reduced recurrences.

Answer 7

The vaginal cylinder applicator is most commonly used. Cylinders come in a variety of diameters (2–4 cm) and lengths to better conform to the patient's anatomy. The cylinder should closely fit to the superior aspect of the vaginal cuff and contact the lateral surfaces of the vagina.

Answer 8

The largest diameter cylinder that can reasonably fit for the patient should be used. The larger cylinder provides a more uniform dose distribution as the diameter of the cylinder increases.

Question 9

What is the typical target length for the treatment of endometrial cancer?

Question 10

Can high-dose-rate (HDR) brachytherapy be used as a boost for treatment of endometrial cancer?

Question 11

What is the prescription dose most commonly used for treatment of endometrial cancer?

Question 12

What are the organs at risk for high-dose-rate (HDR) treatment of endometrial cancer?

Answer 9

The target is typically defined to encompass the dome of the vagina. Most patients have the upper one-half of the vagina treated.

Answer 10

Depending on the extent of myometrium invasion, radiation therapy may include external beam and brachytherapy boost (often considered for more than 50% invasion) or brachytherapy alone (less than 50%).

Answer 11

For high-dose-rate (HDR) brachytherapy, a regimen of three fractions of 7 Gy (21 Gy total dose) to 0.5 cm depth is commonly used. The dose for the brachytherapy may vary when combined with external beam dose.

Answer 12

The bladder, rectum, and sigmoid colon are the organs at risk.

Question 13

What are the tolerance doses to the bladder and rectum for combined external beam and high-dose-rate (HDR) treatment of endometrial or cervical cancer?

Question 14

How can a multichannel vaginal cylinder help in reducing dose to the bladder or rectum?

Question 15

What is the advantage of using volumetric imaging such as CT or MRI compared with the use conventional radiography?

Question 16

What is the International Commission for Radiation Units and Measurements (ICRU) recommendation for specifying the dose to the bladder and rectum?

Answer 13

In equivalent dose of 2 Gy per fraction (EQD2) target coverage D90 should equal 100% of prescription. D2cc to the sigmoid <75 Gy; D2cc to the rectum <75 Gy and D2cc to the bladder <95 Gy should be achieved.

The American Brachytherapy Society consensus guidelines. *Brachytherapy*. 2012;11:33–57.

Answer 14

The multichannel vaginal cylinder is a variation of the standard vaginal cylinder. The applicator contains a central channel and six to eight peripheral channels along the surface of the cylinder. The multichannel cylinder increases the dosimetric control with differential loading of the channels, resulting in an isodose distribution that reduces the dose to the bladder and rectum while maintaining the target dose. A standard cylinder with one central catheter provides only a circular isodose distribution. Another variant is a shielded cylinder, which allows for the insertion of shields in any of the four quadrants of the cylinder to reduce dose to that quadrant.

Answer 15

While localizing and reconstructing source positions based on radiographic markers is simple and accurate, radiographs cannot show soft tissue such as the tumor, the rectum or bladder. Only volumetric imaging modalities can visualize soft tissues and provide three-dimensional characterization of the dose distribution with respect to targets and normal structures.

Answer 16

To provide a bladder calculation point, a Foley balloon is placed in the bladder and filled with ~7 cm^3 of contrast. The bladder dose point is located at the posterior aspect of the balloon. The rectal dose point is located 0.5 cm beyond the posterior vaginal wall.

Question 17

What are the optimization methods for vaginal cylinder treatment planning?

Question 18

When is interstitial brachytherapy used for GYN patients?

Question 19

What high-dose-rate (HDR) brachytherapy option is available for inoperable endometrial cancer?

Answer 17

Optimization adjusts the individual dwell times such that the resultant dose distribution best conforms to the target volume. Optimization points, one for each source dwell position, are typically placed 0.5 cm from the lateral surface of the vagina, and additional optimization points may also be placed at the vaginal apex. Without optimization the dose distribution is oval (left figure), being hotter in the middle of the cylinder's length. Optimization reduces the source dwell times in the middle, and increases them at the ends of the cylinder. This produces a more rectangular dose distribution (right figure). Also shown are the dwell positions (dots), dose points (crosses), and clinical target volume (CTV) (dashed line).

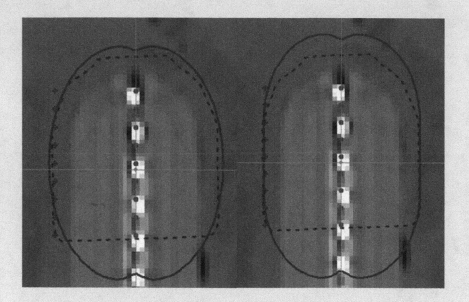

Answer 18

Endometrial and cervical cancers that relapse after surgery in and around the vaginal cuff area with a depth greater than 5 mm can be treated with interstitial brachytherapy. Since there is no uterus a tandem can't be used and the vaginal cylinder can only treat up to 5 mm depth. Three dimensional treatment planning is recommended with CT scan and/or MRI. The treatment plan should be optimized to conform to the clinical target volume and should reduce the dose to critical organs, including the rectum, bladder, urethra, and sigmoid colon.

Answer 19

Medically inoperable endometrial cancer may have a double tandem placed for a boost component of therapy or for palliative intent. The treatment isodose distribution should cover the outer surface of the uterus and give an adequate dose to the gross disease.

Question 20
What brachytherapy treatment techniques can be used for accelerated partial-breast irradiation (APBI)?

Question 21
What patients are not suitable for accelerated partial-breast irradiation (APBI)?

Question 22
What are the available balloon sizes in the balloon-based irradiation?

Question 23
What structures should be contoured for planning balloon-based accelerated partial-breast irradiation (APBI)?

Answer 20

The typical brachytherapy treatment techniques for accelerated partial-breast irradiation include: multiplanar interstitial catheter implant and balloon-based treatment.

Answer 21

1. Age <50 y
2. Positive lymph nodes
3. No lymph nodes examined
4. Tumor size >3 cm
5. Pure ductal carcinoma in situ (DCIS) >3 cm
6. Tumor, node, metastasis (TNM): T3 disease

ABS and ASTRO consensus guidelines. *Brachytherapy*. 2011;10:479–485.

Answer 22

1. Single lumen
   4 to 5 cm, filled with 34 to 70 cc of contrast liquid
   5 to 6 cm, filled with 70 to 125 cc of contrast liquid
2. Ellipsoidal 4 × 6 cm, filled with a maximum of 65 cc of contrast liquid
3. Multilumen 3.5 to 5 cm, filled with 23 to 61 cc of contrast liquid

Answer 23

1. Applicator—balloon surface
2. External—skin surface
3. Lung or the closest ribs
4. Air or seroma within 1 cm from of the applicator

Question 24

What additional structures should be generated for the planning objectives and included in the treatment plan document?

Question 25

What are the geometric and dosimetric parameters relevant to accelerated partial-breast irradiation (APBI)?

Question 26

What is the dose prescription and treatment delivery timeline for accelerated partial-breast irradiation (APBI) high-dose-rate (HDR) brachytherapy?

Question 27

How many dwell positions and prescription points are used for a single-lumen accelerated partial-breast irradiation (APBI) treatment plan?

Answer 24

1. Chest wall—nonbreast tissue
2. Planning target volume (PTV) = 1 cm expansion of the balloon excluding chest wall/ribs, beyond skin
3. PTV for dose evaluation (PTV_EVAL) = PTV - balloon
4. Skin Max—maximum dose of the skin

Answer 25

1. The conformity between the tissue and balloon
2. The symmetry of the balloon within 2 mm of expected dimensions
3. The volume of trapped air/fluid inside seroma <10% of the PTV_EVAL volume
4. The minimum balloon to skin distance >7 mm and max skin dose <145% of the prescription dose (multilumen >5 mm and max <125%)
5. The minimum balloon to chest wall distance >7 mm and max chest wall dose <145% of prescription dose (multilumen >5 mm and max <125%)
6. The physical geometry of the single-lumen balloon should not deviate 2 mm from the expected dimensions

NSABP B-39/RTOG 0413

Answer 26

1. Treatment begins within 9 weeks of lumpectomy or re-excision of margins
2. Prescription dose of 34 Gy, with at least 90% of the prescription dose covering 90% of the PTV_EVAL
3. Two fractions per day, each of 3.4 Gy, separated by at least 6 hours
4. Five treatment days (over a period of 5 to 10 days), a total of 10 fractions and 34 Gy

Answer 27

For a single lumen one dwell point in the center of balloon and two prescription points at the distance from the center of the radius of the balloon + 1 cm. For better coverage and conformity more dwell points can be used, which can create a nonsymmetric dose distribution, based on prescription points on a surface 1 cm beyond the balloon.

Question 28

How many dwell positions are used for a multilumen accelerated partial-breast irradiation (APBI) treatment plan and how is the plan prescribed?

Question 29

What are the acceptable dose volume endpoints for the breast tissue in accelerated partial-breast irradiation (APBI) plans?

Question 30

How is balloon based accelerated partial-breast irradiation (APBI) treatment verified?

Question 31

A brachytherapy balloon is inflated to a radius of 2 cm and an Ir-192 source is positioned at the center. 340 cGy is prescribed to 1 cm depth beyond the surface of the balloon. A second fraction is given without recognizing that the balloon leaked and has a new diameter of 3 cm. What percent of first fraction dose to the surface of the balloon is received at the balloon surface with the second fraction?

Question 32

What are the techniques and applicators used in brachytherapy treatment of cervical cancer?

Answer 28

Depending on the balloon volume, there are typically seven to nine dwell points available in each lumen. The APBI plan is normalized to the target points on the surface of the planning target volume (PTV). With inverse planning, objectives for conformity, coverage and homogeneity, as well as skin and chest wall sparing can be optimized.

Answer 29

The actual volume of tissue receiving 150% (V150) and 200% (V200) of the prescribed dose should be limited to 50 mL and 10 mL, respectively.

Answer 30

To assure integrity of the balloon throughout treatment, an ultrasound or projection X-ray is acquired prior to each fraction and evaluated for any change in the balloon diameter or orientation. These parameters should be compared with those obtained from the treatment plan. For the multilumen treatment, additional care must be taken to check the rotation of the balloon.

Answer 31

Dose fall off for an iridium source is governed by the inverse square law. If the surface of the balloon is 2 cm from the source and is reduced to 1.5 cm from the source the dose will increase by a factor of $2^2/(1.5)^2 = 1.78 = 178\%$.

Answer 32

An intracavitary approach using a tandem and cylinder, tandem and ovoids or tandem and ring can be used or interstitial needles and template for bulky disease.

Question 33
What is a traditional dose specification point for cervical cancer?

Question 34
How is the point A defined in the planning system?

Question 35
What is a definition of point B?

Question 36
Where is the bladder and rectum dose traditionally determined?

Question 37
What are the recommendations for Image-based volumetric approach to cervical brachytherapy?

Answer 33

Dose is prescribed to point A, which is the major critical point for dose specification of intracavitary brachytherapy. It represents the crossing of uterine artery and ureter forming the paracervical triangle.

Answer 34

The definition is 2 cm superior along the tandem from the external cervical os, and 2 cm lateral to the tandem. Point A is recorded for all tandem based treatments, even when using 3D image-based techniques.

Answer 35

Point B represents the pelvic side wall/obturator nodes. Point B is located 5 cm lateral to midline at the same level as point A. It shows the lateral spread of the radiation dose. Its dose is usually 25% of the point A dose.

Answer 36

The bladder dose point is the most posterior part of an antero–posterior line drawn through the center of the bladder catheter balloon. The rectal dose point is located 5 mm posterior to the posterior vaginal wall, along a line perpendicular to the midpoint of the ring or the ovoids.

Answer 37

1. Image-based volumetric information shall consist of CT, or MRI using contiguous slice acquisition with slice thicknesses <3 mm
2. Organs at risk shall be contoured (including bladder, rectum, and sigmoid)
3. Dose-volume histogram (DVH) information should be used for assessment of coverage of the target and dose to organs at risk.
4. Reporting: Standard parameters reported for consistency and comparison should be the D2cc for the organs at risk; D90 and V100 for tumor.

The American Brachytherapy Society consensus guidelines. *Brachytherapy*. 2012;11:33–57.

9

ADVANCED TREATMENT TECHNIQUES

ANTHONY MAGNELLI, TINGLIANG ZHUANG, AND TOUFIK DJEMIL

Question 1

What are the distinguishing features of intensity modulated radiation therapy (IMRT)?

Question 2

What are the differences between intensity modulated radiation therapy (IMRT) and three-dimensional (3D) conformal radiation therapy?

Question 3

How is intensity modulation achieved in an intensity modulated radiation therapy (IMRT) delivery?

Question 4

For a step-and-shoot intensity modulated radiation therapy (IMRT) delivery what are control points and how do they relate to the number of segments?

Answer 1

IMRT is characterized by delivering beams of nonuniform intensity. This requires each beam to be comprised of multiple segments. These nonuniform intensity profiles, or beam fluences, are determined by an optimization algorithm designed to meet the user-defined planning objectives.

Answer 2

3D conformal radiation therapy uses multiple beams each with a single aperture that either conforms to the target volume or purposely protects the critical structures to produce a conformal isodose distribution. IMRT uses beams with multiple beam apertures. These apertures (or segments) are determined by a computer optimization process, called inverse planning. 3D planning is also referred to as forward planning as the planner shapes the apertures to acheive the target goals, rather than specifying the intended dose for the target, and the computer determining the apertures that best achieve this dose in IMRT inverse planning.

Answer 3

Intensity modulation is achieved through the use of multiple apertures (or segments) formed by a multileaf collimator (MLC). An MLC consists of banks of adjacent leaves that can produce most desired beam apertures. An IMRT beam can be delivered using multiple static apertures (step-and-shoot) or a dynamic aperture (sliding window) in order to achieve intensity modulation.

Answer 4

An IMRT beam is delivered using multiple control points. Each control point specifies a multileaf collimator (MLC) shape and a dose to be delivered between control points. Therefore, each IMRT beam segment contains two control points—one specifying that segment's leaf shape and delivering zero dose, and a subsequent control point with the same leaf shape delivering that segment's dose, thus the term step and shoot. The machine then moves to the next control point with the new segment shape.

Question 5
What is the difference between step-and-shoot (static) and sliding window (dynamic) intensity modulated radiation therapy (IMRT) delivery?

Question 6
What is the difference between gradient search and simulated annealing optimization?

Question 7
What is the purpose of performing patient specific intensity modulated radiation therapy quality assurance (IMRT QA)?

Question 8
How are intensity modulated radiation therapy (IMRT) deliveries verified prior to treatment?

Answer 5

A step-and-shoot IMRT plan contains multiple static multileaf collimator (MLC) apertures. The beam is off while the leaves are travelling from one shape to the next. A dynamic sliding window plan delivers dose while the MLC leaves are in continuous motion. Because of the mechanical speed limit on MLCs (a typical maximum mechanical leaf speed is about 2.5 cm/s to 4.0 cm/s specified at the isocenter), dose rate in sliding window delivery varies to prevent the MLC leaf speed exceeding this speed limit.

Answer 6

A gradient search method optimizes the intensity modulated radiation therapy (IMRT) fluence by calculating the gradient of the objective function (or cost function), but this method may result in choosing a plan that resides in a local minimum—that is, the best overall plan may not be achieved. Simulated annealing uses a probabilistic approach, which may choose an optimization path with a higher cost function value in the hopes of finding one later with the global minimum cost value: the best optimized plan.

Answer 7

Patient-specific IMRT QA verifies that the dose computed by the treatment planning system is the same as that delivered by the machine. The QA also verifies that the plan is deliverable by the machine—that is, the plan does not exceed any of the machine's physical limitations.

Answer 8

Patient specific IMRT quality assurance (QA) is performed by delivering the IMRT treatment to a phantom to verify plan deliverability, point dose, and two dimensional (2D) dose distribution accuracy. Measurements are taken using an ion chamber and film, an electronic detector array, or using electronic portal imagers.

Question 9

What are some advantages and disadvantages of treating intensity modulated radiation therapy (IMRT) using a compensating filter rather than multileaf collimator (MLC)?

Question 10

How is the over-travel distance for a multileaf collimator (MLC) defined? How does this affect intensity modulated radiation therapy (IMRT) field size?

Question 11

What is volumetric modulated arc therapy (VMAT)?

Question 12

What precautions should be taken when using intensity modulated radiation therapy (IMRT) to treat a moving target?

Answer 9

Compensating filters can be more robust than MLC-based IMRT since they do not rely on precision of moving leaves and software communication to produce the desired result. They can provide a continuous spectrum of intensity levels. However, the delivery of compensator-based IMRT plans are very labor intensive to produce and require significant therapist effort as each beam will require a different compensator to be placed in the head of the linear accelerator (linac).

Answer 10

The over-travel distance is the maximum distance that a leaf tip can extend beyond the isocenter. A typical distance is 10 cm. If this distance is smaller than half the maximum field size, then this will limit the usable field size available for an IMRT beam.

Answer 11

VMAT is a form of intensity modulated radiation therapy (IMRT) using rotating beams called arcs. These arcs are delivered with variable gantry speed, dose rate, and multileaf collimator (MLC) leaf speed in order to create the desired dose distribution. VMAT plans are created using inverse planning to generate the required MLC motion patterns that are synchronized to the gantry angle and dose rate.

Answer 12

The motion of a target may have an interplay effect with the motion of the multileaf collimator (MLC) leaves. This effect can be alleviated by using a smaller number of apertures and a larger aperture size. Motion management techniques can also be employed to minimize target motion. These may include abdominal compression, voluntary or active breathing control, or respiratory gating.

Question 13
What is multileaf collimator (MLC) interplay?

Question 14
How is intensity modulation achieved in a proton beam?

Question 15
What is the difference between direct aperture optimization and traditional two-step intensity modulated radiation therapy (IMRT) optimization?

Question 16
Which treatment modality typically uses more monitor units (MUs) to deliver the same dose: three-dimensional (3D) conformal or intensity modulated radiation therapy (IMRT)?

Answer 13

When intensity modulated radiation therapy (IMRT) is delivered, it is only irradiating part of the target at a time. It is easy for a moving target to move out of this small aperture, or have the wrong part of it irradiated. Since the planning system does not model tumor motion, the dose delivered to the moving target may differ substantially from the planned dose distribution. In a three-dimensional (3D) plan, the whole tumor is being irradiated at once. As a result, tumor motion is not as important.

Answer 14

Proton beams are modulated using specially milled compensators that modulate beam intensity by using varying thickness. Photon intensity modulated radiation therapy (IMRT) can also be compensator based, but this is no longer common, as it requires the therapist to enter the treatment vault for each beam to change the compensator. This is also a limiting factor in the number of beams used for proton therapy. More recent proton units are using scanning pencil-beam techniques to deliver intensity modulation.

Answer 15

Direct aperture optimization (DAO) incorporates multileaf collimator (MLC) leaf positions during inverse optimization. Users define the number of allowable apertures per beam or per plan directly. Traditional two-step IMRT first optimizes an idealized (or continuous) fluence, and then converts this fluence into a machine deliverable MLC sequence by accounting for MLC leaf size, leakage, and minimum aperture size, which reduces the conformality of the idealized plan.

Answer 16

IMRT typically requires more MUs to deliver the same dose than 3D conformal. IMRT beams are comprised of several apertures, each smaller than a single, large aperture used for a 3D conformal plan. In order to deliver the same dose across the entire field using smaller apertures, more total MUs are typically required. For some 3D conformal plans, especially when a 60° physical wedge is used, the 3D conformal plan may have higher MUs than the IMRT plan.

Question 17

Comparing intensity modulated radiation therapy (IMRT) and three dimensional (3D) conformal plans for the same treatment, what is the typical increase in monitor unit (MU)?

Question 18

What is a downside of intensity modulated radiation therapy (IMRT) delivery compared with conventional radiation therapy?

Question 19

Between volumetric modulated arc therapy (VMAT) and intensity modulated radiation therapy (IMRT), which typically uses more monitor units (MUs) to deliver the same dose?

Question 20

What are common intensity modulated radiation therapy (IMRT) objective types used for targets?

Answer 17

The typical increase in MU is a factor of 2 to 3 for IMRT versus 3D conformal plans, depending on the delivery method and optimization method used. Methods such as direct aperture optimization (DAO) result in a smaller increase in MU.

Answer 18

Because IMRT deliveries use an increase number of monitor units (MUs), there is more leakage present from the linear accelerator (linac) head and therefore higher dose delivered outside the intended treatment area. There is also an integral dose increases with IMRT.

Answer 19

VMAT uses fewer monitor units than conventional two-step IMRT plans. This is because VMAT apertures are more open. It is possible for VMAT plans to have higher MU than the conventional IMRT plans for cases with overlapping targets and organs at risk, requiring small treatment apertures.

Answer 20

Objectives used for target volumes are those that require the target to receive a minimum dose or higher. This can be achieved by defining a minimum point dose (Min dose), or minimum dose received to a certain volume (Min dose volume histogram [DVH]). To control the dose distribution within the target, the target may be required to receive a specific uniform dose or a maximum dose.

Question 21

What are common intensity modulated radiation therapy (IMRT) objective types used for organs at risk (OAR)?

Question 22

What sites are not typical candidates for intensity modulated radiation therapy (IMRT) and why?

Question 23

How is an objective function used to optimize an intensity modulated radiation therapy (IMRT) plan?

Question 1   9.2 STEREOTACTIC RADIATION THERAPY

What are the defining characteristics of a stereotactic body radiation therapy (SBRT) treatment?

Answer 21

Objectives used for OAR are those that require the OAR to receive a maximum dose or lower. This can be achieved by defining a maximum point dose (Max dose), or maximum dose received to a certain volume (Max dose volume histogram [DVH]).

Answer 22

Targets that undergo significant intra-fraction motion during treatment are typically not considered ideal candidates for IMRT due to the motion interplay effect. This effect can be alleviated by reducing the number of total overall segments, and increasing the minimum allowed aperture size. Additionally, sites with large tumor volume such as abdominal cancers are often equally well treated with three-dimensional (3D) conformal.

Answer 23

The objective function is formulated as follows. For a given set of machine parameters (leaf shapes, monitor units [MU]), the squared difference between each stated objective dose and its current calculated dose is computed. Each squared difference is also multiplied by a user defined weighting factor. The objective function is the sum of these individual weighted squared differences. The optimization algorithm searches for the minimum of the objective function, by varying the machine parameters.

Answer 1

SBRT treatments are usually given in five fractions or less. Treatment plans are designed to give a highly conformal dose to the target with very steep dose falloff and heterogeneous dose distribution within the target.

Question 2

What sites are commonly treated with stereotactic body radiation therapy (SBRT)?

Question 3

What differences in dose distribution are expected between coplanar and noncoplanar deliveries?

Question 4

What are the tumor volume dose and cord constraints for a stereotactic body radiation therapy (SBRT) spine treatment according to Radiation Therapy Oncology Group (RTOG) 0631?

Question 5

What planning margin is applied to stereotactic body radiation therapy (SBRT) spine targets?

Answer 2

Lung, spine, liver, pancreas, prostate, and adrenal.

Answer 3

Noncoplanar plans can achieve higher conformality and steeper dose gradients.

Answer 4

RTOG 0631 prescribes a dose of 16 Gy to the tumor. Cord dose is limited to a maximum dose of 14 Gy to 0.03 mL of the contoured cord volume, and <10% of the contoured cord volume receiving 10 Gy. Contoured cord volume is the length of the spinal cord 5 to 6 mm above and below the tumor volume level.

RTOG 0631. Phase II/III Study of Image-Guided Radiosurgery/SBRT for Localized Spine Metastasis

Answer 5

There is no margin added to the gross tumor volume for either presumed microscopic extension of disease or for setup error.

Question 6

What is an internal target volume (ITV)?

Question 7

What are typical clinical target volume (CTV) and planning target volume (PTV) expansions in lung stereotactic body radiation therapy (SBRT)?

Question 8

What image guidance techniques are employed in stereotactic body radiation therapy (SBRT)?

Question 9

What imaging studies are used for CT simulation for liver stereotactic body radiation therapy (SBRT)?

Answer 6

When a target will be moving during treatment, it is useful to define a volume that encompasses this motion. This is called the ITV. It can easily be derived from contouring the target in each phase of the 4DCT (4-dimensional computed tomography, which is a type of CT acquisition which can visualize a target through its range of motion). The ITV is then the volume that covers each phase's target contour. Only the breathing phases used for treatment should be used for determining the ITV.

Answer 7

Following the guidelines of Radiation Therapy Oncology Group (RTOG) 0813, PTV expansion in SBRT is less than in conventional radiation therapy (RT). If breathing excursion is observed using 4DCT, a 5-mm PTV expansion is added to the internal target volume (ITV). If free breathing CT is acquired with no ITV, the gross tumor volume (GTV) is expanded 1 cm in the superior-inferior direction and 5 mm in the axial plane. No CTV expansion is typically created for SBRT treatments.

Answer 8

Common techniques include cone-beam CT (CBCT) and stereoscopic X-rays.

Answer 9

CT scans with and without contrast are required for liver SBRT. Contrast studies are used to aid in tumor visualization. Contrast-free studies are required for CT-based planning to avoid incorrect effective depth due to the presence of the high density contrast agent.

Question 10

How is a stereotactic frame used to target intracranial lesions?

Question 11

What are the advantages and disadvantages of frameless versus frame-based intracranial stereotactic radiosurgery (SRS)?

Question 12

What types of patient immobilization devices are common for stereotactic body radiation therapy (SBRT) treatment?

Question 13

What types of treatment delivery are used for stereotactic body radiation therapy (SBRT)?

Answer 10

The patient is scanned with a stereotactic head-frame affixed to the skull. The head-frame provides a coordinate system in which the target position is referenced. The head-frame is subsequently attached to the couch for treatment delivery.

Answer 11

Frameless SRS increases patient comfort since it does not require the frame to be affixed directly to the skull. It also allows for simulation and planning to take place on a different day from treatment. However, it also increases the risk of intra-fraction motion and increased uncertainty in target localization.

Answer 12

For lung or abdominal treatments, vacuum fitted blue bags or alpha cradles are used to reproducibly position patients for treatment. Vacuum-affixed plastic wrap can provide additional restriction if desired. For cranial or upper spinal treatments, a thermoplastic mask system is commonly used.

Answer 13

Noncoplanar three-dimensional (3D) conformal beams, conformal arc, intensity modulated radiation therapy (IMRT) and volumetric-modulated arc therapy (VMAT) deliveries are all common techniques for SBRT.

Question 14
How can rectal uncertainty be minimized for a prostate stereotactic body radiation therapy (SBRT)?

Question 15
What are the differences between conformal arc therapy and dynamic conformal arc therapy?

Question 16
What is the difference between dynamic conformal arc therapy and volumetric-modulated arc therapy (VMAT)?

Question 17
What is a typical lung constraint for a lung stereotactic body radiation therapy (SBRT) treatment?

Answer 14

A rectal balloon can be inserted and inflated to a reproducible volume during simulation and treatment. The balloon serves to both immobilize the prostate and to position the rectum reproducibly. The balloon can be inflated with air or water. Water ensures the volume of the balloon is the same each time, but air allows for better sparing of the rectal wall.

Answer 15

Conformal arc therapy is a rotational treatment modality that uses a fixed beam aperture. During dynamic conformal arc therapy, the beam aperture will change its shape to conform to the projected tumor volume as the gantry rotates around the patient. This requires dynamic multileaf collimator (MLC) support.

Answer 16

Multileaf collimator (MLC) leaves will move during treatment delivery for both dynamic conformal arc therapy and VMAT. However leaf motion in dynamic arc therapy is determined by the projection of the tumor volume. For VMAT, inverse planning determines multileaf collimator (MLC) position at each gantry angle.

Answer 17

The typical lung constraint is lung V20 <10% according to Radiation Therapy Oncology Group (RTOG) 0813.

Question 18

Is intensity modulated radiation therapy (IMRT) a permissible treatment technique for lung stereotactic body radiation therapy (SBRT)?

Question 19

What magnetic resonance imaging (MRI) sequences are used for stereotactic body radiation therapy (SBRT) spine treatment planning?

Question 20

What is the advantage of using the average of a four dimensional computed tomography (4DCT) acquisition versus a free breathing CT for lung stereotactic body radiation therapy (SBRT)?

Question 21

What is the dose constraint for liver in stereotactic body radiation therapy (SBRT)?

Answer 18

IMRT can be used for SBRT of slow moving lung tumors. IMRT in SBRT lung is more frequently used for central tumors, due to the importance in sparing critical structures. The number of fractions for central lung tumors is typically 5 versus 1 to 3 fractions for noncentral lung tumor locations.

Answer 19

T1 and short TI inversion recover (STIR) sequences are used for target volume and spinal cord delineation.

Answer 20

When using cone-beam CT (CBCT) for image guidance, the pretreatment CBCT will bear more resemblance to the average CT due to the slow acquisition of the CBCT.

Answer 21

Based on the Radiation Therapy Oncology Group (RTOG) 1112 trial, 700 mL of liver should be spared to less than 15 Gy.

RTOG 1112. Randomized Phase III Study of Sorafenib versus Stereotactic Body Radiation Therapy followed by Sorafenib in Hepatocellular Carcinoma

Question 1   **9.3 RESPIRATORY MANAGEMENT**

How is respiratory motion assessed?

Question 2

What techniques are available for respiratory management?

Question 3

What is gated treatment?

Question 4

What are commonly used gating windows?

Answer 1

Respiratory motion can be assessed by using fluoroscopy or four dimensional computed tomography (4DCT).

Answer 2

Respiratory management can be achieved by using abdominal compression, active breathing control, voluntary breath hold, or respiratory gating.

Answer 3

Gated treatments use a surrogate signal to indicate the position of the tumor. This could be surface trackers, strain gauge belt or a spirometer. A certain range of this signal is then selected by the user to indicate when the tumor is at the desired treatment position. This signal will then be used to activate the treatment beam when the signal falls within the user-defined window.

Answer 4

Gating windows commonly include exhale or inhale phases, or the 30% to 70% respiratory phases. Left breast or chest wall therapy will use end inhale to increase the distance between the heart and the target. Lung therapy can use end exhale, as this is a repeatable position for the tumor, or end inhale to improve the dosimetric parameters of the normal lung.

Question 5

What are some commonly used surface trackers for respiratory motion?

Question 6

What are some advantages and disadvantages of gated treatment techniques?

Question 7

What is active breathing coordination (ABC)?

Question 8

How can the reproducibility of active breathing coordination (ABC) be verified?

Answer 5

The Varian real-time position management (RPM) system uses an infrared reflector placed on the patient's chest and an infrared (IR) camera to observe and record the breathing motion. BrainLab ExacTrac also uses infrared markers placed directly on the patient's body for this purpose. VisionRT/optical surface mapping uses a video camera to render the patient's body surface directly, which is used as a motion surrogate.

Answer 6

Gated treatments enable treatment of the target during only a portion of its range of motion, minimizing the size of the treatment volume and potentially minimizing normal tissue toxicity. Gated treatments also provide an alternative motion management technique for patients who may not be able to tolerate breath hold, abdominal compression, or other more restrictive methods. However, gated treatments typically take longer to deliver than normal treatments. Additionally, the assumption that the surrogate signal accurately reflects the position of the internal tumor volume may not be true in all cases.

Answer 7

ABC is a device used to hold the patient's breathing cycle at a predetermined threshold. It comprises a mouth piece with a spirometer. The flow of air is stopped once the threshold amount of air has been inhaled.

Answer 8

ABC reproducibility can be verified by observing the patient under fluoroscopy while the ABC is in use. Additionally, multiple CT scans can be acquired and fused in order to assess residual motion.

Question 1

How many bits are in one byte?

Question 2

How many bytes are needed to express a floating point value?

Question 3

How long does it take to transmit a CT dataset consisting of 115 slices, each with 512×512 pixels and a bit depth of 32 bits over a network connection of 100 Mbit/s?

Question 4

What is recorded by a record and verify system?

Answer 1

There are 8 bits in one byte. Then there are kilo (10^3), Mega (10^6), and Giga (10^9) bytes. A CT is around 100 MB, a cone-beam CT (CBCT) around 30 MB, a radiation therapy (RT) plan file is 10 to 100 kB.

Answer 2

A floating point number contains a sign (positive or negative) 23 numbers representing it, and 8 numbers representing its exponent, for example, $-1.2345 = -1 \times 12345 \times 10^{-4}$. 4 bytes are required to express a floating point value.

Answer 3

Size of the image is:

$512 \times 512 \times 32$ bits/image $\times 115$ images $= 9.65 \ 10^8$ bits

Time to transmit is size divided by network speed

$9.65 \ 10^8 / 10^8$ bit/s $= 9.65$ s

Answer 4

A record and verify system records the actual aspects of treatment delivery such as gantry angle, monitor units (MU), collimator and jaw settings, and all other major machine settings. Treatment verification images such as portal images and cone-beam CT (CBCT) scans are also stored. Additionally, patient demographic information and treatment plan details may be included.

Question 5
What is digital imaging and communication in medicine (DICOM)?

Question 6
What is the file structure of a digital imaging and communication in medicine (DICOM) image file?

Question 7
What is digital imaging and communication in medicine-radiation therapy (DICOM-RT)?

Question 8
What is a PACS and what is its purpose?

Answer 5
DICOM is a file standard used for the communication and storage of medical imaging.

Answer 6
DICOM files contain a data and header section. The data section contains the image data itself. The header contains information such as patient name, medical record number, birthdate, scan date and time, image acquisition parameters, and other pertinent details.

Answer 7
DICOM-RT is an extension of the DICOM standard specific to radiation oncology applications. DICOM-RT contains seven specifically designed DICOM objects—RT Image, RT Structure Set, RT Plan, RT Dose, RT Beams Treatment Record, RT Brachy Treatment Record, and RT Treatment Summary Record.

Answer 8
PACS stands for Picture Archiving and Communication System. Its purpose is to provide a secure digital repository for all medical images used for patient care.

10

SPECIALIZED TREATMENT

YVONNE PHAM AND GENNADY NEYMAN

Question 1

What is the mechanical tolerance for the radiosurgery devices?

Question 2

What are the main characteristics of stereotactic radiosurgery (SRS)?

Question 3

What are the main features of stereotactic radiosurgery (SRS) plans?

Question 4

What types of radiation beams are used for stereotactic radiosurgery (SRS)?

Answer 1

Less than or equal to 1 mm.

Klein, EE, et al. Task Group 142 report: quality assurance of medical accelerators. *Med Phys.* 2009;36(9):4197–4212.

Answer 2

Stereotactic radiosurgery requires three-dimensional (3D) imaging, stereotactic targeting, steep dose gradients, and high accuracy of beam delivery.

Answer 3

High prescription doses per fraction and high degree of dose conformality.

Answer 4

Gamma-rays, megavoltage X-rays, and heavy-charged particles.

Question 5

What is the definition of conformity index (CI) in radiosurgery?

Question 6

Which factors contribute to a sharp dose penumbra in linac-based stereotactic radiosurgery (SRS)/ stereotactic body radiation therapy (SBRT) using circular cones and arcs?

Question 7

What is a typical quality assurance test used for linac-based radiosurgery?

Question 8

How does the Gamma Knife work?

Answer 5

The volume covered by the prescription isodose line divided by the volume of the target. The closer to one, the better the conformity is. This ratio should be ≤2. This index does not imply target coverage, which must be confirmed separately.

Answer 6

Multiple noncoplanar arcs, 4 to 6 MV beam energy, small collimator-to-tumor distance.

Answer 7

A Winston–Lutz test. A rod with a small ball bearing (bb) is attached to the treatment couch. The bb is placed at isocenter and images are taken with the linac beam at multiple gantry, collimator, and couch angles. The images are checked to ensure the bb remains in the center of the image, which ensures the isocenter is fixed with respect to motion of the gantry, collimator, and couch.

Lutz W, Winston KR, Maleki N. A system for stereotactic radiosurgery with a linear accelerator. *Int J Radiat Oncol Biol Phys.* 1988;14(2):373–381.

Answer 8

The Gamma Knife contains 192 (Perfexion model) or 201 (B, C, and 4C models) cobalt-60 sources. The Perfexion is arranged in a cone shape with eight individual sectors and the B, C, and 4C models are arranged in hemispherical array and housed in a heavily shielded unit. Radiation is precisely collimated to deliver the high dose of radiation to the designated target(s) while sparing the surrounding tissues. Complex-shaped lesions can be treated by combining varying-sized collimators with selected sector/beam blocking and dose weighting using very sophisticated computer planning software.

Question 9

Which factors contribute to a sharp dose penumbra in Gamma Knife radiosurgery?

Question 10

What is the definition of the inhomogeneity index in radiosurgery?

Question 11

Which isotope is used in Gamma Knife radiosurgery and what is its average energy and half-life?

Question 12

What is a typical time between changing the cobalt-60 (Co-60) sources for Gamma Knife radiosurgery?

Answer 9

The very large number of noncoplanar isocentric beams (192 for Perfexion model, 201 for earlier models) and small collimator-to-target distance. The geometric penumbra is inversely proportional to source to collimator distance thus moving the collimator closer to the surface of the patient decreases the geometric penumbra.

Answer 10

The ratio of the maximum dose to the prescription dose of the target. This ratio should be ≤ 2.

Answer 11

Cobalt-60 (Co-60), average energy of 1.25 MeV (one gamma of 1.17 and one of 1.33 MeV). The half-life of Co-60 is 5.26 years.

Answer 12

About one half-life of cobalt-60 (Co-60), so between 5 and 6 years for a source exchange. The initial dose rate is around 3 Gy/min.

Question 13

Describe a typical Gamma Knife procedure.

Question 14

Who must sign the Gamma Knife plan before treatment delivery?

Question 15

What agency regulates a Gamma Knife machine?

Question 16

What diseases and doses are treated in Gamma Knife stereotactic radiosurgery (SRS)?

Answer 13
1. Daily QA of the system
2. Attachment of the stereotactic frame to the patient's head
3. Stereotactic imaging using high resolution MRI, CT, or angiogram as required
4. Localization of the images in the Gamma Knife frame of reference
5. Delineation of the target volumes
6. Dose planning and evaluation of the dose plans with all members of the radiosurgery team
7. Treatment delivery
8. Removal of the frame

Answer 14
The neurosurgeon, radiation oncologist, and a medical physicist; all of whom must be trained for Gamma Knife procedures.

Answer 15
Since the Gamma Knife uses cobalt-60, which is made in a nuclear reactor (by-product material), its use is regulated by the Nuclear Regulatory Commission (NRC) or the State Departments of Health for the Agreement States.

Answer 16

Tumor/Disorder	Dose (Gy)
Meningioma	13–14
Pituitary adenoma	Nonsecretory: 14–16 Secretory: 18–25
Vestibular Schwannoma	12–13
Arteriovenous Malformation	14–27
Trigeminal Neuralgia	80–90 (to 100% isodose line)
Brain Metastases	
2 cm or less	20–24
2.1–3 cm	18
3.1–4 cm	15

Question 17

What are the advantages and disadvantages of Gamma Knife versus linac-based stereotactic radiosurgery (SRS)?

Question 18

What special equipment and imaging is required for linac-based stereotactic radiosurgery (SRS)?

Question 19

When might fractionated stereotactic radiosurgery (SRS) be preferable to single session radiosurgery?

Answer 17

Type	Main Advantages	Main Disadvantages
Gamma Knife	High accuracy and precision; Less moving parts—easier QA; Used for about 50 years—much experience; Reliability of the machine—little down time	Brain only; Usually single session only; Can be used for multifractionation with Extend but no image-guided radiation therapy (IGRT) capabilities; Needs to change sources in 5–6 years; Radiation safety precautions
Linac-based SRS	Single or fractionated treatments; image-guided radiation therapy (IGRT) capabilities; Treatment of extracranial sites	With a heavy gantry, it is more difficult to maintain SRS required tolerance; Time needed for QA; Different manufacturers—more difficult to generalize collected data

Answer 18

1. High definition multileaf collimators (MLC) (leaf width of 2.5 mm) or circular cones with diameters from 4 to 30 mm
2. Image-guidance systems like planar X-ray based, cone-beam CT (CBCT), optical, or ultrasound-based
3. Electronic portal image detectors (EPID) or films

Answer 19

1. For brain tumors with maximum dimension more than 4 cm
2. For lesions that are located very near to critical organs like optic apparatus, the full clinical dose to the target cannot be achieved without exceeding max safe dose of organ-at-risk (OAR).
3. For retreatments

Question 1

What is total body irradiation (TBI)?

Question 2

Why is total body irradiation (TBI) used and what is the typical dose range used?

Question 3

What is the most common prescription in total body irradiation (TBI)?

Question 4

Where is the dose prescription point usually located for anterior–posterior and posterior–anterior (AP/PA) fields with stationary photon beams for total body irradiation (TBI)?

Answer 1

TBI is a special radiotherapeutic technique, which delivers to a patient's whole body a uniform dose to within ±10% of the prescribed dose.

Answer 2

It is used as a conditioning regimen for hematopoietic stem cell transplantation. TBI can serve to eradicate any residual cancer and immunosuppress the host so that it cannot reject the allogeneic donor stem cells. 2 to 15 Gy is the typical dose range that is used in conjunction with chemotherapy.

Answer 3

12 Gy delivered in six 2 Gy fractions at two fractions per day (separated by minimum of 6 hours) over 3 days.

Answer 4

It is an intercept between two lines from midsagittal to midaxial and midcoronal to midaxial planes. This is usually close to midplane at the umbilicus.

Question 5

For total body irradiation (TBI), what is the purpose of a spoiler screen that is placed in front of the patient?

Question 6

How is field size typically maximized for total body irradiation (TBI)?

Question 7

What dose rate is typically used for total body irradiation TBI?

Question 8

What photon energies are typically used for total body irradiation (TBI)?

Answer 5

A spoiler brings the surface dose to at least 90% of the prescribed dose. Typically, an acryclic spoiler screen of 1 to 2 cm thickness, dependent on beam energy, is placed 10 cm in front of the patient.

Answer 6

By treating the patient at an extended source to skin distance (SSD) of 300 to 400 cm and turning the collimator to 45° the field size can be maximized. This results in field sizes greater than 2 m for a 40×40 cm^2 collimator.

Answer 7

The dose rate should be less than 0.1 Gy/min to minimize side effects. A low-dose-rate is an additional benefit of treating at extended source to skin distance (SSD). Using the inverse square rule, a 2 Gy/min dose rate at 100 cm SSD is reduced to 0.125 Gy/min at 400 cm SSD.

Answer 8

6 MV photons are typically used with parallel opposed TBI fields if the patient's thickness is <35 cm and the source to skin distance (SSD) is at least 300 cm. If the patient is >35 cm in thickness, energies higher than 6 MV photons should be used in order to minimize excessively high doses to the subcutaneous tissues compared to the midpoint dose. Recall that the effective energy [percent depth dose (PDD)] of a photon beam increases with increasing SSD.

Question 9

What techniques are used to account for tissue heterogeneity in the thoracic region during total body irradiation (TBI)?

Question 10

What measurements are typically performed to estimate the lung dose?

Question 11

What typical techniques can be used for total body irradiation (TBI)?

Question 12

What is total skin irradiation (TSI)?

Answer 9

The lungs are a critical dose-limiting structure in TBI. Lungs have a lower density and receive a dose that exceeds the prescribed dose by 10% to 24%, depending on what energy beams are used. Lung blocks are typically used to reduce dose to the lungs to 80% of the prescription dose.

Answer 10

Thermoluminescence dosimeters (TLDs), diodes, or metal oxide semiconductor field effect transistors (MOSFETs) can be placed on the patient anterior to the lung for irradiation with or without blocks to estimate the lung dose. The thickness or number of fractions where blocking is needed to achieve a safe lung dose is then determined.

Answer 11

1. Anterior–posterior and posterior–anterior (AP/PA) technique with patient standing in upright position at extended source to skin distance (SSD)
2. Patients lying down on the floor in supine and prone positions (20 cm away from the floor) while the gantry swings from 320° to 40°
3. A bilateral technique—treating with left/right lateral opposing fields with patient seated on the couch in a semi-fetal position.

Answer 12

TSI is a technique using electrons in the energy range of 2 to 9 MeV for treating superficial lesions covering large areas of the body.

Question 13
What is total skin irradiation (TSI) used for, and what is the typical prescription dose?

Question 14
What is the Stanford technique for total skin irradiation (TSI)?

Question 15
Why are two beams used for each patient orientation?

Question 16
What areas are shielded when a patient undergoes total skin irradiation (TSI)?

Answer 13

TSI is used for large lesions extending to about 1 cm depth, like mycosis fungoides or other cutaneous lymphomas with typical prescription doses of 30 to 40 Gy.

Answer 14

It is a six field technique (anterior–posterior [AP], posterior–anterior [PA], and four obliques) positioned 60° apart around the circumference of the patient with each field consisting of two component beams at some angle (15°) to the horizontal plane. The patient stands in three of six positions per day.

Answer 15

This is done to reduce the X-ray contamination hitting the patient and to provide a large electron beam with sufficient dose uniformity in the vertical dimensions.

Answer 16

Typically the eyes and nails are shielded since these areas would otherwise receive a higher dose than the rest of the skin after 20 Gy.

Question 17
What areas are typically boosted?

10.3 PARTICLE THERAPY

Question 1
What are the most common heavy charged particles used in radiation therapy?

Question 2
What are heavy ions?

Question 3
What are some typical heavy ions that can be used for radiation therapy?

Answer 17

Typically the soles of the feet, vertex of the head, perineum, and medial thighs are boosted. These areas are not fully exposed to the total skin irradiation (TSI) beams.

Answer 1

Protons, heavy ions, and negative pions. Electrons are also charged particles, but are not considered heavy particles. Neutrons are heavy particles, but are not charged.

Answer 2

Heavy ions are medium to large Z atoms that have been stripped of all their electrons. They generally do not change direction significantly while traveling through matter due to their large mass.

Answer 3

Neon, argon, and carbon.

Question 4

What is the typical energy range for heavy ion beams used for radiation therapy?

Question 5

Why is carbon considered the optimum heavy ion for radiation therapy?

Question 6

What are negative pions?

Question 7

How are negative pions produced?

Answer 4

400 to 500 MeV/nucleon. It is the kinetic energy/nucleon that determines the range of a heavy ion, not the total kinetic energy of the ion. For example, a carbon ion has a Z of 6 (the number of protons) and typically 6 neutrons, so 12 nucleons. The kinetic energy of the carbon ion would therefore have to be 4,800 MeV, to achieve the therapy energy of 400/MeV.

Answer 5

The stopping power of a charged particle is dependent on Z^2. For ions that have a Z greater than carbon, their linear energy transfer (LET) values are too large and can result in biological damage to tissues before reaching their target. Also, carbon ions do not fragment as much as other ions when they collide directly with nuclei within a medium. The nuclear fragments could deliver dose beyond the Bragg peak, which is unwanted.

Answer 6

Pi mesons, or pions, are approximately 15% of the mass of a proton and thus scatter three times as much as protons given their lower mass. A negative pion exhibits a usual Bragg curve but has the additional unique property of getting captured by a nucleus of the medium when it comes to rest which results in release of kinetic energy due to nuclear fragmentation and subsequently enhances the dose near the Bragg peak region.

Answer 7

They are produced using 400 to 800 MeV protons that hit a beryllium target.

Question 8
What is the typical energy and range for radiation therapy for negative pions?

Question 9
How do protons interact through a medium?

Question 10
What is the typical energy range for proton therapy?

Question 11
How are protons for therapy produced?

Answer 8

A typical energy is 100 MeV and the range is 24 cm in water.

Answer 9

Protons mainly interact with atomic electrons and nuclei of the medium through the Coulomb force. These interactions involve inelastic collisions of protons with atomic electrons where proton kinetic energy is lost to produce excitation and ionization of atoms, resulting in absorbed dose.

Answer 10

Proton beams used for radiation therapy typically have energies in the range of 150 to 250 MeV. This creates a Bragg peak at 15 to 40 cm deep in water.

Answer 11

The source of protons is usually hydrogen gas. These protons are then accelerated in cyclotrons or synchrotrons, both circular accelerators, where the proton repeatedly passes through the same accelerating cavities, kept in path by magnetic fields. The strength of the magnetic field depends on the charge of the proton, its mass, velocity, and the radius of curvature of the accelerator.

Question 12

What is the relative biologic effectiveness (RBE) of protons for treatment planning purposes?

Question 13

What is the Bragg peak?

Question 14

Why do electrons not exhibit a Bragg peak?

Question 15

What is the spread-out Bragg peak (SOBP) and how is it useful?

Answer 12

In order to help evaluate clinical response to proton versus photon beams, most facilities use an RBE factor of 1.1 for protons. The RBE varies with energy and is greatest and likely higher than 1.1 in the region of the Bragg peak.

Answer 13

The Bragg peak is the peak in dose deposition at the end of the range for a heavy charged particle. For monoenergetic proton beams, the depth–dose curve is initially fairly flat with a slow increase in dose with depth, followed by a sharp increase of dose near the end of the range. As the proton loses energy traveling in a medium, it slows down and the rate of energy loss per unit path length increases. The rate of energy loss is maximal as the particle velocity reaches zero at the end of its range. The depth of the Bragg peak increases as the energy of the initial proton beam increases.

Answer 14

While electrons do lose more energy as they slow down, they are prone to scattering easily and do not follow a straight track like heavy charged particles. This removes the possibility of seeing a Bragg peak with depth. There would be a Bragg peak as a function of electron track length.

Answer 15

SOBP involves using a combination of proton beams energies to help cover a wider depth of coverage than the peak of one energy alone. Higher energy beams help cover the distal end of the target volume while lower energy beams cover the proximal portion.

Question 16

How can a spread-out Bragg peak (SOBP) be produced?

Question 17

Compared to photons, do inhomogeneities cause a larger or smaller effect on dose distribution for protons?

Question 18

Can a CT be used directly for proton treatment planning?

Question 19

What does robust planning mean in proton therapy?

Answer 16

The proton energy must be modulated to create a SOBP. There are typically two ways to do this. The first method is to use a rotating variable thickness filter that may be called a "modulation wheel" made of variable thicknesses of acrylic glass or graphite, which degrades the beam energy. As the beam travels through the variable thickness filter, a Bragg peak of a precalibrated range is created. The second method is to change the beam energy with the proton accelerator.

Answer 17

Larger. Tissue inhomogeneities can change attenuation per unit distance by only a few percent for photons compared to proton beams where tissue inhomogeneities drastically change the range of the beam, which could cause critical structures to be over-irradiated while tumors may be under-irradiated. This is important not just in planning, but with inter- and intrafraction changes in inhomogeneity such as tumor motion in the lung.

Answer 18

Current CT units use X-rays instead of protons to create their image. Thus, it is necessary to convert CT numbers to proton stopping powers to calculate the proton range required for the treatment field. This can be done by employing a calibration curve that is unique to the CT scanner and kVp used and takes into account electron density and the composition of tissues. There are errors and uncertainties in the conversion of CT numbers to relative proton stopping power, in particular two materials may have the same CT number, but different relative proton stopping power. These uncertainties are taken into account during the treatment planning process by adding proximal and distal margins on each treatment field to attain the intended spread-out Bragg peak (SOBP).

Answer 19

Robust planning or optimization takes into account several proton-specific uncertainties including the distal and proximal margins along the beam axis, lateral field edges, and conversion of CT numbers to proton stopping power. These uncertainties are especially important at tissue interfaces of differing density and composition. Corrective techniques to help account for these uncertainties have been utilized such as computing dose distributions at the higher and lower end of these uncertainties to ensure complete coverage of the target volume. Monte Carlo calculation algorithms are utilized to help improve calculation accuracy.

Question 20

How does the lateral (perpendicular to central axis) dose gradient compare to the central axis of the beam for proton beams?

Question 21

What are some disadvantages of proton beams?

Question 22

What are some types of neutron therapy?

Question 23

What energy neutrons are used?

Answer 20

The lateral dose gradient is broader. As the proton beam loses energy, there is a lateral broadening of the beam near the end of range due to multiple scattering in the medium.

Answer 21

There may be beam contamination from other particles, particularly neutrons that have a much higher biological effect on tissue and can affect dose distributions. Also, the accelerator used to produce protons is much larger than a photon machine and has high initial and maintenance costs.

Answer 22

One type of therapy is external beam neutron therapy, which is created by accelerated protons or deuterons striking a beryllium target. A second type is called boron neutron capture therapy (BNCT). This therapy consists of administration of Boron-10 (B-10), which will preferentially concentrate into tumor cells, followed by irradiation of the tumor site by neutrons. This method takes advantage of a transmutation reaction where the B-10 nucleus absorbs a neutron to become an unstable nucleus, which subsequently emits a short-range alpha particle and a lithium ion that deposit their energy within the cell containing the original B-10 atom. The combined path length of both resulting particles is approximately one cell diameter, which helps to confine the treatment to a tumor cell while sparing normal cells.

Answer 23

Protons or deuterons are typically accelerated using cyclotrons to energies of about 50 MeV, which strike a beryllium target and produce neutron beams that are energetically equivalent to a 6-MV X-ray beam.

Question 24

What sites have been treated with neutrons?

Question 25

What are the disadvantages of neutron therapy?

Question 1

What is hyperthermia?

Question 2

What is the typical desired treatment temperature for hyperthermia?

Answer 24

Minor and major salivary gland neoplasms are commonly treated by neutrons. Other sites where neutrons have been utilized but not shown to have a clear advantage compared to photon and electron therapy include other head and neck tumors, malignant gliomas, soft-tissue sarcomas, and prostate cancer.

Answer 25

Neutrons can have various interactions with the medium resulting in the emission of gamma rays, recoil protons, alpha particles, heavy charged particles, and neutrons. This broad spectrum of secondary radiation from neutron interactions results in a broad penumbra, making it more difficult to collimate and plan the beam arrangement. Also, energy absorption from neutron therapy does not correlate smoothly as a function of neutron energy; there are spikes or resonance peaks where large amounts of absorption may occur at variable neutron energies.

Answer 1

Hyperthermia is a type of treatment in which tissues in the body are exposed to higher than normal temperatures. The idea behind hyperthermia treatment is that increased temperature in cancer cells cause them to become more sensitive to radiation therapy and/or chemotherapy, thus it is used in combination with these modalities.

Answer 2

41°C to 45°C.

Question 3

What is the type of electromagnetic energy used for hyperthermia?

Question 4

How long is a typical hyperthermia treatment?

Question 5

Is hyperthermia alone an effective treatment?

Question 6

When should radiation therapy be administered if hyperthermia is being used?

Answer 3

Microwave energy is used, typically around 915 MHz to give up to a 2 cm depth of heating.

Answer 4

A typical treatment lasts for 60 minutes.

Answer 5

Hyperthermia is almost always used as an adjunctive treatment to radiation or chemotherapy. Hyperthermia alone may result in a transient tumor response, but no long-term tumor control has been reported.

Answer 6

Hyperthermia is typically given for 60 minutes and followed by a radiation treatment within an hour of completion. Hyperthermia is typically given two to three times each week. An enhancement is still seen if hyperthermia is given directly after radiation as well.

Question 7

What sites are most often treated with hyperthermia?

Question 8

What is the thermal enhancement ratio?

Question 9

What phase of the cell cycle is most sensitive to hyperthermia?

Answer 7

Locally recurrent breast cancers, malignant melanomas, and head and neck cancers are the most frequently treated sites with hyperthermia in conjunction with radiation therapy. Randomized trials have also revealed a benefit to hyperthermia in combination with radiation for other cancers including esophagus, bladder, cervical, rectal, bladder, glioblastoma multiforme, and sarcoma.

Answer 8

The thermal enhancement is the ratio of radiation dose to produce a specified biologic effect *without heat* to the dose of radiation needed for equivalent effect *with heat*.

Answer 9

Late S phase; this is also the phase of the cell cycle most resistant to X-rays and thus results in the synergistic effects of radiation and hyperthermia when used in combination.

11

QUALITY

PENG QI AND ANTHONY MAGNELLI

Question 1   11.1 THERAPY EQUIPMENT QUALITY ASSURANCE

How frequently is quality assurance (QA) on a linear accelerator (linac) performed?

Question 2

What is the protocol used to perform the absolute output calibration of a linear accelerator (linac)?

Question 3

What are the accepted tolerances for linear accelerator (linac) output deviation measured during daily, monthly, and annual quality assurance (QA)?

Question 4

How strictly are photon and electron beam profile flatness and symmetry required to be maintained?

Answer 1

Linac QA requires daily, monthly, and annual QA procedures, and whenever a repair or change is made that affects the function of the linac.

Answer 2

The absolute output calibration of a linac defines the relationship of the radiation dose deposited in the tissue with the output of the machine (measured in arbitrary monitor units [MUs]). The procedure of this calibration in water is performed using the American Association of Physicists in Medicine (AAPM) task group (TG)-51 protocol. The TG-51 protocol prescribes the use of ion chambers and electrometers, which have been calibrated at an accredited dosimetry laboratory in a cobalt-60 beam. The user then uses a conversion factor, k_Q, to convert from cobalt-60 to the quality of the beam being calibrated.

Almond PR, et al. AAPM's TG-51 protocol for clinical reference dosimetry of high-energy photon and electron beams. *Med Phys*. 1999; 26:1847–1870.

Answer 3

The annual linear accelerator (linac) calibration procedure for photon and electron beams must be performed by a qualified medical physicist and the absolute dose measured in water according to the American Association of Physicists in Medicine (AAPM) task group (TG)-51 protocol must be within 1% of the nominally defined output (typically 1.0 cGy/MU).

The monthly output verification must be within 2% of the nominal defined output for each beam energy. The daily output verification must be within 3% of the nominally defined output for each beam energy.

Klein EE, et al. Task Group 142 report: quality assurance of medical accelerators. *Med Phys*. 2009;36:4197–4212.

Answer 4

The constancy checks of photon and electron beam flatness and symmetry in monthly quality assurance (QA) procedure are to be within 1% of the baseline value. The same 1% tolerance is required for annual QA, but a range of field sizes should be checked.

Klein EE, et al. Task Group 142 report: quality assurance of medical accelerators. *Med Phys*. 2009;36:4197–4212.

Question 5

How is a new high-dose-rate (HDR) source calibrated?

Question 6

How accurate are the treatment couch position indicators required to be?

Question 7

What are the daily quality assurance (QA) procedures performed on a CT simulator?

Question 8

What additional quality assurance (QA) tests are performed monthly and annually on a CT simulator?

Answer 5

The activity of high-dose-rate brachytherapy sources must be verified by a qualified medical physicist prior to clinical use. Source activity must be measured by using a calibrated well-type ionization chamber and electrometer. Activity of the source must be within 5% of the manufacturer's specified activity.

Kutcher GJ, et al. Comprehensive QA for radiation oncology: report of AAPM Radiation Therapy Committee Task Group 40. *Med Phys*. 1994;21:581–618.

Answer 6

Treatment couch position accuracy is very important due to automated positioning controlled by image-guided radiation therapy (IGRT) systems. Couch positioning accuracy is required to be within 2 mm/1° for machines used for conventional treatments, and 1 mm/0.5° for machines used for stereotactic body radiation therapy (SBRT) and stereotactic radiosurgery (SRS) treatments.

Klein EE, et al. Task Group 142 report: quality assurance of medical accelerators. *Med Phys*. 2009;36:4197–4212.

Answer 7

According to task group (TG)-66, consistency of the CT number in water, image noise, spatial integrity, and orthogonality of lasers with the imaging plane must be checked daily. Additional checks of the accuracy of laser isocenter marking are common.

Mutic S, et al. Quality assurance for computed-tomography simulators and computed-tomography-simulation process: report of the AAPM Radiation Therapy Committee Task Group No. 66. *Med Phys*. 2003;30:2762–2792.

Answer 8

According to the American Association of Physicists in Medicine (AAPM) task group (TG)-66, monthly QA includes tests for image quality (such as uniformity, noise, CT number accuracy, contrast, and spatial resolution), mechanical components including table orientation and motion, and safety issues. For annual QA, extra tests include radiation profile, imaging dose, and electron density to Hounsfield unit (HU) calibration.

Question 9
What are the acceptable criteria for agreement between the light field and radiation field?

Question 10
How often is the electron beam energy required to be verified, and what is its tolerance?

Question 11
What are the daily quality assurance (QA) procedures performed on a high dose rate (HDR) machine?

Question 12
How is a linear accelerator (linac) quality assurance (QA) for a stereotactic body radiation therapy (SBRT)/stereotactic radiosurgery (SRS) machine different from that of a machine used primarily for conventional therapy?

Answer 9

According to the American Association of Physicists in Medicine (AAPM) task group (TG)-142 guidelines, the field sizes defined by the light and radiation should be in agreement within 1 mm or 1% per field side for modern asymmetric jaws.

Klein EE, et al. Task Group 142 report: quality assurance of medical accelerators. *Med Phys*. 2009;36:4197–4212.

Answer 10

Each electron beam energy is verified monthly and annually. Electron beam energy is checked monthly by measuring doses at two different depths to spot check the percent depth dose (PDD) of the beam, and must agree within 2% or 2 mm. Annually, electron R50 values are required to be measured to within 1 mm. The electron beam quality specifier, R50, is defined as the depth at which the electron beam percent depth dose is 50% of its maximum.

Almond PR, et al. AAPM's TG-51 protocol for clinical reference dosimetry of high-energy photon and electron beams. *Med Phys*. 1999;26:1847–1870.

Answer 11

The daily QA includes checks for timer accuracy, source position accuracy, door interlocks, source exposure indicators, video and intercom system, radiation monitoring system and devices, and control console function.

Wilkinson DA. High dose rate (HDR) brachytherapy quality assurance: a practical guide. *Biomed Imaging Interv J*. 2006;2:e34.

Answer 12

According to the American Association of Physicists in Medicine (AAPM) task group (TG)-142 guidelines, the tolerance of QA for a linear accelerator (linac) used for SBRT/SRS is more stringent than for a machine used primarily for conventional therapy.

Procedure	Conventional Tolerance	SBRT/SRS Tolerance
X-ray monitor units (MU) linearity	±2% ≥ 5 MU	±2% ≥ 5 MU, ±5% (2–4 MU)
Radiation and mechanical Isocenter coincidence	±2 mm	±1 mm
Lasers	1.5–2 mm	1 mm
Collimator size indicator	2 mm	1 mm
Couch position	2 mm/1°	1 mm/0.5°
Imaging accuracy	≤2 mm	≤1 mm

Klein EE, et al. Task Group 142 report: quality assurance of medical accelerators. *Med Phys*. 2009; 36:4197–4212.

Question 13

What monthly tests should be performed for cone-beam CT (CBCT) imaging systems?

Question 14

How frequent is the quality assurance (QA) performed for cone-beam CT (CBCT) imaging-guidance systems?

Question 15

One qualified radiation therapist did daily output measurement. If the result exceeds the baseline by 5%, what actions should be triggered?

Question 16

How frequently is multileaf collimator (MLC) quality assurance (QA) performed?

Answer 13

Monthly quality assurance (QA) for CBCT system comprises imaging and treatment coordinate coincidence, imaging safety interlocks and imaging quality tests such as geometric distortion, spatial resolution, contrast, Hounsfield unit (HU) constancy, and uniformity and noise.

Klein EE, et al. Task Group 142 report: quality assurance of medical accelerators. *Med Phys*. 2009;36:4197–4212.

Answer 14

For linear accelerators (linacs) equipped with CBCT systems, the QA for CBCT imaging verification should be performed daily, monthly, and annually. The daily QA tests the typical image-guided radiation therapy (IGRT) process of imaging and shifting the patient.

Klein EE, et al. Task Group 142 report: quality assurance of medical accelerators. *Med Phys*. 2009;36:4197–4212.

Answer 15

If this level is exceeded, no further treatment should be given until a radiation oncology physicist has discovered the source of the discrepancy. If the output difference is in the range of 3% and 5%, then treatment may continue at the discretion of the radiation oncology physicist.

Kutcher GJ, et al. Comprehensive QA for radiation oncology: report of AAPM Radiation Therapy Committee Task Group 40. *Med Phys*. 1994;21:581–618.
Klein EE, et al. Task Group 142 report: quality assurance of medical accelerators. *Med Phys*. 2009;36:4197–4212.

Answer 16

According to the American Association of Physicists in Medicine (AAPM) task group (TG)-142 guidelines, the MLC QA should be performed weekly, monthly, and annually.

Klein EE, et al. Task Group 142 report: quality assurance of medical accelerators. *Med Phys*. 2009;36:4197–4212.

Question 17

What is the tolerance of the quality assurance (QA) test for multileaf collimator (MLC) position repeatability?

Question 18

For step-and-shoot or dynamic-arc (volumetric modulated arc therapy [VMAT]) delivery multileaf collimator (MLC), are the quality assurance (QA) procedures similar?

Question 19

What quality assurance (QA) procedures are performed on treatment planning systems (TPS)?

Answer 17

According to the American Association of Physicists in Medicine (AAPM) task group (TG)-142 guidelines, the tolerance for leaf position repeatability is ±1 mm. The test is normally performed using a "picket fence"–like test pattern (see following figure). This test irradiates multiple bands created by the leaves that should be neither over- or underlapping if the leaves move correctly.

Klein EE, et al. Task Group 142 report: quality assurance of medical accelerators. *Med Phys*. 2009;36:4197–4212.

Answer 18

Because continuous gantry and MLC leaf motion are involved during VMAT delivery, additional tests should be performed for VMAT delivery MLC. Those tests include leaf speed tests, picket-fence test at different gantry angles and delivery of specialized VMAT fields to test synchronization of gantry speed, dose rate and leaf position.

Klein EE, et al. Task Group 142 report: quality assurance of medical accelerators. *Med Phys*. 2009;36:4197–4212.

Answer 19

Both dosimetric and nondosimetric elements of the TPS must be tested. The tests include reviewing the system change and error logs, system input/output devices (eg, CT input) and dose calculation. Tests are performed daily, monthly, annually and after any upgrade to the TPS.

Fraass B, et al. American Association of Physicists in Medicine Radiation Therapy Committee Task Group 53: quality assurance of clinical radiation therapy treatment planning. *Med Phys*. 1994;25:1773–1829.

Question 20

What is an end-to-end test?

Question 21

What are the periodic quality assurance (QA) procedures on CT images in treatment planning systems (TPS)?

Question 22

What are the quality assurance (QA) procedures on plan evaluation (dose-volume histogram) in treatment planning systems (TPS)?

Question 23

What are periodic quality assurance (QA) procedures on dose calculation for treatment planning systems (TPS)?

Answer 20

An end-to-end test checks the entire radiation therapy system. It starts with the CT of a specialized phantom, on which an isocenter is marked. The CT is sent to the treatment planning systems (TPS) and planned. The plan is then sent to the linear accelerator (linac). The phantom is placed according to the isocenter marks, and port films taken to ensure the fields planned match the shapes within the phantom. In the case of Radiation Therapy Oncology Group (RTOG) credentialing, the plan is delivered to the phantom which contains film and thermoluminescence dosimeters (TLDs). The dose measured is then compared to the plan to confirm accuracy of delivering the planned dose.

Answer 21

Because the majority of radiation therapy dose calculation is CT-based calculation, it is important to perform periodic QA on CT images. Those tests include CT scan transfer, CT geometry and CT number (related to the electron density of the tissue) check.

Fraass B, et al. American Association of Physicists in Medicine Radiation Therapy Committee Task Group 53: quality assurance of clinical radiation therapy treatment planning. *Med Phys*. 1994;25:1773–1829.

Answer 22

These tests include plan normalization, relative and absolute dose, volume determination, histogram dose bin size, calculation of grid size and points distributions, consistency in structure and dose statistics.

IAEA TRS 430. Commissioning and quality assurance of computerized planning systems for radiation treatment of cancer. *IAEA*. 2004.

Answer 23

For treatment planning systems the most critical issue is the accuracy and consistency of dose and monitor units (MU) calculation. The following tests are recommended by Technical Report Series (TRS) 430: (a) calculated dose per beam; (b) beam weighting; (c) summed dose distribution; (d) plan normalization; and (e) MU calculations.

IAEA TRS 430. Commissioning and quality assurance of computerized planning systems for radiation treatment of cancer. *IAEA*. 2004.

Question 24

What is acceptance testing for a medical linear accelerator?

Question 25

What is required for commissioning for a medical linear accelerator?

Question 1   11.2 PATIENT SAFETY

What is the new patient safety initiative launched jointly by the American Society of Radiation Oncology (ASTRO) and the American Association of Physicists in Medicine (AAPM)?

Question 2

Where can you find guidelines to follow in making decisions regarding patient safety issues?

Answer 24

Performed by a qualified medical physicist, the acceptance testing ensures the machine meets the specifications of the manufacture and of the purchase agreement. The tests include a number of safety, mechanical, and dosimetric checks. The safety checks (door interlocks, emergency stops, and survey of exposure levels in the treatment control area), should be done before other tests to ensure a safe environment for the testers.

Kutcher GJ, et al. Comprehensive QA for radiation oncology: report of AAPM Radiation Therapy Committee Task Group 40. *Med Phys*. 1994;21:581–618.

Answer 25

The process of commissioning a linear accelerator involves a comprehensive and accurate measurement of all dosimetric parameters to completely describe the radiation beams. This information is then used to model the accelerator in the treatment planning system. Annually, measurements are taken to confirm the radiation beams still conform to the original commissioning data. If it does not conform, the treatment planning systems (TPS) beam model will have to be updated.

Das IJ, et al. Accelerator beam data commissioning equipment and procedure: report of the TG-106 of the Therapy Physics Committee of the AAPM. *Med Phys*. 2008;35:4186–4215.

Answer 1

The Radiation Oncology Incident Learning System™ (RO-ILS) was launched in 2014. RO-ILS documents, analyzes and tracks patient safety-related incidents submitted by participating Radiation Oncology centers.

Answer 2

Task group (TG) reports from the American Association of Physicists in Medicine (AAPM), white papers from ASTRO, the American College of Radiology (ACR)/ASTRO accreditation and practice standards, and government regulations (eg, 10 Code of Federal Regulations (CFR) part 20).

Question 3
What agency regulates reactor-produced materials?

Question 4
Who regulates naturally occurring radioactive materials and X-ray machines?

Question 5
What safety measures must be included in the practice of radiation oncology?

Question 6
Given the routine use of cone-beam CT (CBCT)-based image verification, what are the current designs to avoid mechanical injury by the machine?

Answer 3

The Nuclear Regulatory Commission (NRC) regulates the reactor-produced materials such as cobalt-60 (Co-60). States can choose to adopt the NRC regulations and become agreement states.

Answer 4

Individual states regulate these forms of radiation.

Answer 5

a. A treatment management system for prescription, treatment parameters setup and delivery, and daily dose recording and summation
b. A physics program for calibrating equipment that ensures accurate dose delivery to the patient
c. A system for independent verification of treatment parameters (external beam) by another qualified person or method before the first treatment
d. A system for the radiation oncologist and medical physicist to independently check all relevant brachytherapy practice parameters to be used prior to each procedure
e. A program to prevent mechanical injury by the machine or accessory equipment
f. Visual and audio contact with the patient while under treatment
g. A policy requiring two forms of patient identification as well as verification of treatment parameters prior to each treatment

ACR-ASTRO Practice Parameter for Radiation Oncology Revised 2014, available at http://www.acr.org/guidelines

Answer 6

A mechanical system, a protection ring attached to the gantry with springs, is used on Elekta linear accelerators (linacs), and a laser detection system is installed on current Varian machines (laser guard). In addition, the kV and MV image panels have interlocks, which will stop the gantry motion when the force applied on the panel exceeds the preset limits. Based on the pre-CBCT couch positions, the Varian control system can move the couch to a "safe zone" before the image acquisition to avoid potential collisions. The couch will be restored to its initial position after the CBCT imaging. Despite these safety designs, it is recommended that radiation therapists perform a dry run to check the possible mechanical injury to the patient from the machine.

Question 7

Which two forms of patient identification are commonly used in radiation oncology?

Question 8

What quality assurance (QA) checks should be performed in radiation oncology? Among the QA checks, which individual check is the most effective for detecting potential errors?

Question 9

Among the members of the treatment team, who can declare a "time-out"?

Question 10

Is it necessary to implement the checklist procedure in the practice of radiation oncology?

Answer 7

A common combination of patient identification is a patient's full name and date of birth. An identification wristband or face photo can also be used.

Answer 8

QA checks that should be performed include physician plan review, physics plan review, therapist chart review, pretreatment intensity-modulated radiation therapy (IMRT) QA, Chart rounds, timeout by therapist, source-to-surface distance (SSD) check, port films, online CT, in vivo dosimetry, and physics weekly checks. Physics plan review is more sensitive than other individual checks.

Ford EC, Terezakis S, Souranis A, et al. Quality control quantification (QCQ): a tool to measure the value of quality control checks in radiation oncology. *Int J Radiat Oncol Biol Phys.* 2012;84:e263–e269.

Answer 9

Each member of the treatment team (including therapists, physicists, physicians, etc.) should have a right to declare a time-out if he or she has a concern or question regarding the plan and treatment during the course of the treatment.

Hendee WR. Herman MG Improving patient safety in radiation oncology. *Prac Radiat Oncol.* 2011:16–21.

Answer 10

Yes. Studies have shown that the use of medical checklist reduces the likelihood of errors in medical practice.

Gawande A. *The Checklist Manifesto: How to Get Things Right.* New York, NY: Metropolitan Books; 2009.

Question 11

Why is patient specific intensity-modulated radiation therapy (IMRT) quality assurance (QA) necessary?

Question 12

What are the action levels for patient specific intensity-modulated radiation therapy (IMRT) quality assurance (QA)?

Question 13

What are the recommendations for the treatment of patients with implanted cardiac pacemaker?

Question 14

A patient has been diagnosed with cervical carcinoma and has decided to start radiation therapy. What will happen with her pregnancy?

Question 15

A pregnant patient needs to undergo whole brain radiation therapy. What are the recommendations when you simulate and port the patient?

Answer 11

Based upon the American College of Radiology (ACR) guidelines, the accuracy of dose delivery must be documented for each course of treatment by irradiating a phantom that contains either calibrated film to sample the dose distribution or an equivalent measurement system (such as an ion chamber or diode array) to verify that the dose delivered is the dose planned.

ACR-ASTRO practice parameter for intensity modulated radiation therapy (IMRT) Amended 2014 (Resolution 39).

Answer 12

The action levels can vary based upon the type of treatment, disease site, measurement device, delivery method, etc. Typically, the action level for the absolute point dose difference between the planned and measured dose is ± 5%. Comparing the measured and planned dose distribution is typically achieved with a gamma index, where a >90% of passing rate using 3%/3 mm criteria is required. For stereotactic body radiation therapy (SBRT), the action levels can be more stringent than conventional IMRT treatment.

Low DA, et al. A technique for the quantitative evaluation of dose distributions. *Med Phys*. 1998;35:879–887.

Answer 13

The American Association of Physicists in Medicine (AAPM) task group (TG)-34 recommends limiting accumulated dose to the pacemaker to 2 Gy. Individual manufacturers may, however, have lower limits. It is also a good practice to avoid using photon beams with energy above 10 MV, to remove neutrons, which may directly damage the electronics of the pacemaker. There is an active task group (TG)-203 formed by AAPM to update the information regarding this issue.

Marback JR, et al. Management of radiation oncology patients with implanted cardiac pacemakers: report of AAPM Task Group No. 34. *Med Phys*. 1994; 21:85–90.

Answer 14

According to the Nuclear Regulatory Commission (NRC) 10 Code of Federal Regulations (CFR) Part 20.1208, the dose equivalent to the embryo/fetus should not exceed 5 mSv during the entire pregnancy. Doses below 0.1 Gy should be safe, with doses up to 0.5 Gy not necessarily fatal, depending on the stage of the pregnancy, but would result in fetal damage. Treatment of cervical cancer is not compatible with preservation of the fetus.

Kal HB, Struikmans H. Radiation therapy during pregnancy: fact and fiction. *Lancet Oncol*. 2005;6:328–333

Answer 15

Following the As Low as Reasonably Achievable (ALARA) principle, one should conduct a CT scan with large slice thickness (eg, >5 mm), short scan range along the superior-inferior direction, and low kVp and/or mAs. When doing portal imaging, a single exposure portal image is recommended.

Question 16

According to the Nuclear Regulatory Commission (NRC), who should be included in the radiation safety committee to oversee the use of byproduct material at a medical institution?

Question 17

For stereotactic body radiation therapy (SBRT) treatments, should a radiation oncologist be present at the start of each treatment, prior to irradiation?

Question 18

According to the Nuclear Regulatory Commission (NRC), what are the components of a written directive?

Question 19

What is the dose limit used for the Nuclear Regulatory Commission (NRC) 10 Code of Federal Regulations (CFR) part 35 (report and notification of a medical event)?

Question 20

If a medical event is discovered, how soon should a licensee notify the Nuclear Regulatory Commission (NRC) by phone?

Answer 16

The committee should include the authorized user, the radiation safety officer (RSO), a nurse, and a representative of management who is neither an authorized user nor an RSO.

Answer 17

Yes. Before each treatment, the radiation oncologist must be present to verify the integrity of the patient setup and patient positioning using image guidance.

Solberg TD, Balter JM, Benedict SH, et al. Quality and safety considerations in stereotactic radiosurgery and stereotactic body radiation therapy. *Prac Raidat Oncol*. 2011 (white paper).

Answer 18

A written directive is required for source-based procedures (brachytherapy, gamma knife and other source-based teletherapy). Depending on the type of application (high dose rate [HDR], low dose rate [LDR], permanent or temporary), the directive must contain: the dosage (and fractionation if applicable), route of delivery, radionuclide, number of sources and total source strength, treatment site, and the patient's name. This must be signed by the authorized user physician.

Answer 19

The dose limit is 0.05 Sv (5 rem) effective dose equivalent, 0.5 Sv (50 rem) to an organ or tissue, or 0.5 Sv (50 rem) shallow dose equivalent to the skin.

Answer 20

According to NRC 10 Code of Federal Regulations (CFR) 30.3045, a licensee shall notify by phone the NRC operation center no later than the next calendar day after discovery of the event. The licensee shall submit a written report to the appropriate NRC regional office within 15 calendar days after the discovery of the event.

12

RADIATION SAFETY AND REGULATIONS

MIKE STRONGOSKY AND HENRY BLAIR

Question 1

What is the frequency for inventory and survey for a radioactive material storage area, for example, Cs-137?

Question 2

What is the survey limit requirement for a patient's release who has received a radioactive source or radiopharmaceutical?

Question 3

What is the frequency for survey meter calibration?

Question 4

What does *ALARA* stand for?

Turn page to see the answers. **359**

Answer 1

Quarterly, according to Nuclear Regulatory Commission (NRC) rules.

Answer 2

The Nuclear Regulatory Commission (NRC) guidelines are based on keeping the radiation level to a member of the public the patient may interact with below 500 mrem. Therefore, the survey limit is different depending on the source used, a table is provided by the NRC. For I-131 it is <7 mrem/hr and for I-125 it is 1 mrem/hr, both measured at 1 m from the patient surface.

Answer 3

Annually, before the initial use and after any repair.

Answer 4

As Low As Reasonably Achievable. This is the basis of radiation protection planning and accounts for the cost and effort to reduce the risk of radiation to zero.

Question 5

What is the negligible individual risk level (NIRL)?

Question 6

As a radiation worker, if you separately undergo radiation therapy, does this affect your annual dose limit?

Question 7

What is the lifetime limit for a radiation worker?

Question 8

What is equivalent dose?

Answer 5

The National Council on Radiation Protection and Measurements (NCRP) definition of NIRL is "the level of average annual excess risk of fatal health effects attributable to radiation below which efforts to reduce radiation exposure to the individual is unwarranted." The current value is 0.01 mSv.

Answer 6

The 50 mSv per year is an *occupational* dose limit; it does not include radiation from background, medical exposure as a patient, or dose as a member of the general public.

Answer 7

The National Council on Radiation Protection and Measurements (NCRP) limit is 10 mSv multiplied by age in years.

Answer 8

Equivalent dose takes into account the different biological effects of different types of radiation, such as photon, proton, thermal neutrons (<10 MeV), neutrons, and heavy particles. Equivalent dose is the dose in Gy (J/kg) multiplied by the radiation weighting factor (W_R) of the radiation. Its unit is the Sievert (Sv). The old unit was rem, 100 rem = 1 Sv.

Question 9

What are the International Commission on Radiological Protection (ICRP) recommended values for radiation weighting factors W_R?

Question 10

What is effective dose equivalent (EDE)?

Question 11

What are the National Council on Radiation Protection and Measurements (NCRP) values for tissue weighting factors w_T?

Question 12

What is the whole body effective dose equivalent (EDE) limit for a member of the general public?

Answer 9

Types of Radiation	Radiation Weighting Factor
X-ray, Gamma ray, electrons, and beta particles	1
Protons	2
Neutrons	A range from 5 to 20 depending on energy

Answer 10

Just as equivalent dose takes into account the damage of different types of radiation, effective dose takes into account the sensitivity of different tissues, effective dose equals absorbed dose multiplied by the tissue weighting factors. EDE is then the combination of absorbed dose, multiplied by the radiation and tissue weighting factors.

Answer 11

Tissue	Tissue Weighting Factor
Gonads	0.2
Bone marrow, colon, lung, stomach	0.12
Bladder, breast, esophagus, liver, thyroid	0.05
Bone surface, skin	0.01
Remaining tissues (adrenals, brain, small and large intestine, kidney, muscle, pancreas, spleen, thymus, and uterus)	0.05

The sum of the tissue weighting factors is 1, so the effective dose equals the absorbed dose when the body is uniformly irradiated.

NCRP Report 116 Limitation of Exposure to Ionizing Radiation, 1993

Answer 12

1 mSv/y (100 mrem/y), this is determined based on risk compared to other every day hazards.

Question 13

What is the whole body effective dose equivalent (EDE) limit for an occupational worker?

Question 14

What is the effective dose equivalent (EDE) limit for a pregnant occupational worker?

Question 15

What is the dose limit for radiation workers to the eyes and extremities?

Question 16

What types of radiation badges are available?

Answer 13

50 mSv/y (5,000 mrem/y).

Answer 14

5 mSv/term (0.5 mSv/month).

Answer 15

The extremities are limited to 500 mSv/y and the lenses of the eye to 150 mSv/y.

Answer 16

X-ray film, thermoluminescent dosimeter (TLD) badges, and optically stimulated luminescent dosimeter (OSLD). These are available as body and ring badges.

Question 17

What is the average yearly exposure (per person) in the United States from background radiation?

Question 18

What percentage of medical radiation exposure do CT studies account for?

Question 19

What are the Nuclear Regulatory Commission (NRC) requirements for determining if hospital staff needs radiation monitoring badges?

Question 20

What is the purpose of the Conference of Radiation Control Program Directors (CRCPD)?

Answer 17

3.1 mSv, depending on geographic location. The majority of this (2.3 mSv) is from Radon.

Answer 18

Approximately 50%.

Answer 19

The NRC requires monitoring if there is a likelihood of the individual receiving more than 10% of the annual occupational limit and/or having access to areas where the radiation exposure rate could exceed 1 mSv (100 mrem) per hour.

Answer 20

One of the main functions of the CRCPD is to produce suggested state regulations for control of radiation. These are referred to by individual states as guidelines in creating their own regulations governing radiation therapy.

Question 21

Who regulates the transport of radioactive materials?

Question 22

What does the transport index (TI) on a package of radioactive material indicate?

Question 23

What are the requirements (limits) for radioactive material transportation labels: White I, Yellow II, and Yellow III?

Question 24

For each piece of therapy equipment, what information is typically required to be kept?

Answer 21

Department of Transportation.

Answer 22

The highest dose rate at 1 m from the surface. This partially determines the type of label placed on the package, either White I for TI of 0, Yellow II for TI less than 1, or Yellow III otherwise.

Answer 23

Label	Surface Radiation		Radiation at 1 m
White I	<0.5 mrem/h		Not applicable
Yellow II	<50 mrem/h	AND	<1 mrem/h
Yellow III	Exceeds 50 mrem/h	OR	Exceeds 1 mrem/h

Answer 24

(a) Report of acceptance testing.
(b) Records of all surveys, calibrations and periodic QA checks, and names of the people who performed them.
(c) Records of maintenance and/or modifications performed, as well as the names of people who performed such services.
(d) Name and signature of the qualified medical physicist or authorized individual authorizing the return of the therapy equipment to clinical use after any service or intervention that affects patient treatment.

Question 25

What is the American College of Radiology (ACR) recommendation regarding an independent check (second check) of initial dose calculations?

Question 26

What is the typical process for the radiation oncologist checking port films?

Question 27

A medical event (misadministration) for external beam therapy is defined by the calculated weekly administered dose differing from the weekly prescribed dose by more than what percent?

Question 28

A medical event (misadministration) for external beam therapy is defined by the calculated total administered dose differing from the total prescribed dose by more than what percent?

Answer 25

The check shall be conducted before the third fraction or before 20% of the total dose when the treatment schedule provides less than 10 fractions. The independent check includes utilizing another individual or method approved and documented by the medical physicist to verify dose calculations.

Answer 26

Initial port films shall be checked by the radiation oncologist prior to the second treatment and the port films shall be rechecked at least every 10 treatments.

Answer 27

30%.

Answer 28

20%, unless the treatment has three or fewer fractions, in which case the limit is 10%.

Question 29

Besides exceeding the permissible differences between administered and calculated doses; what are the other three ways to define a medical event (misadministration) for external beam therapy?

Question 30

What is the definition of a medical event for radioactive material?

Question 31

After it has been ascertained that a medical event has occurred, what are the time requirements (verbal and written) for reporting it to the regulating body?

Question 32

After initially notifying the regulating body of a medical event (misadministration), how long do you have to notify the referring physician?

Answer 29

Wrong patient, wrong treatment, or wrong treatment site.

Answer 30

Any of the following is a medical event: (a) if one or more sealed sources are leaking; (b) administration of the wrong radioactive drug/material; (c) administration to the wrong individual; (d) administration by the wrong mode of treatment; (e) the delivered dose deviated greater than 20% of the prescription dose.

Answer 31

By telephone no later than the next calendar day (24 hours) and a written report within 15 days.

Answer 32

No later than 24 hours.

Question 33

How long must a record of a medical event (misadministration) be kept?

Question 34

What are the differences between stochastic and nonstochastic (deterministic) effects?

Question 1   **12.2 SHIELDING**

In the equation for primary barrier shielding, $B_p = P(d_{pri})^2/WUT$ where B_p is the thickness of shielding required, identify d_{pri}, P, W, U, T.

Question 2

What is the definition of use factor (U)?

Answer 33

Three years.

Answer 34

Stochastic effects are nondeterministic or random in nature. The severity of damage is independent of the dose, but the probability of a biological effect increases with the dose. An example of a stochastic effect is cancer. There is usually a threshold dose for nonstochastic effects, the severity of which varies with the dose. Examples of nonstochastic effects would be erythema and cataract formation.

Answer 1

P is dose limit per week permitted outside the barrier for protection, d_{pri} is distance in meters from the primary radiation source to point protected, W = workload (expressed in Gy/wk), U = use factor, T = occupancy factor.

Answer 2

Use factor is the fraction of the time per week that the primary beam falls on the barrier. Typical use factors are floor 0.31, walls 0.2, and ceiling 0.26. In the case of secondary barriers, $U = 1$ is assumed due to scattered radiation and head leakage uniformly distributed around the vault.

NCRP Report No 151 Structural Shielding Design and Evaluation For Megavoltage X- and Gamma-Ray Radiation therapy Facilities, 2005.

Question 3

What is the definition of occupancy factor (T)? Give some examples of common occupancy factors.

Question 4

For the dose limit per week permitted outside the barrier for protection (P) in the shielding equation, what is the maximum permissible radiation measured in mR for controlled and noncontrolled areas?

Question 5

In the equation for the secondary barriers to shield against scattered radiation $B_s = Pd^2_{sca} \, d^2_{sec} \, 400/\alpha WTF$ (F = beam size at the patient), what does "α" represent? What is the unit for the distance of d_{sca} and d_{sec}?

Question 6

What is the use factor, U, for secondary barriers?

Answer 3

The fraction of time a particular area will be occupied. Examples: Full occupancy ($T = 1$) offices, laboratories, occupied buildings or living quarters, clinical work stations. Partial occupancy ($T = 1/5$) rest rooms, corridors. Occasional occupancy ($T = 1/20$) waiting rooms, stairways, closets.

NCRP Report No 151 Structural Shielding Design and Evaluation For Megavoltage X- and Gamma-Ray Radiation therapy Facilities, 2005.

Answer 4

A controlled area is for radiation workers so its dose levels are consistent with the dose limits of radiation workers, namely 1 mSv/wk and 50 mSv/y (100 mrem/wk and 5,000 mrem/y). Noncontrolled areas are for the public, and the limits are 0.02 mSv/wk and 1 mSv/y (2 mrem/wk or 100 mrem/y).

Answer 5

Scattered radiation is radiation that scatters from the primary treatment beam. It therefore has a lower energy than the primary beam. "α" is the fractional scatter at 1 m from the scatterer (eg, wall). It depends on angle and field size. At 90° a typical α is 10^{-3} to 10^{-4}. d_{sca} is the distance from the source to the scatter; d_{sec} is the distance from the scatter to the area of interest both measured in meters.

Answer 6

U is 1 because the secondary barriers are always exposed to the scattered radiation and head leakage when the beam is on.

Question 7
Neutrons can be generated above what energy?

Question 8
What is the advantage of using a maze for a radiation therapy vault?

Question 9
What is a TVL?

Question 10
What materials are commonly added to vault doors to help reduce dose from neutrons?

Answer 7

Photon beams of 10 MV and above are capable of producing neutrons by photonuclear reactions, where a high energy photon interacts directly with a nucleus placing it into an excited state, which then decays via neutron emission.

Answer 8

The use of a maze can ease the design of the door. Without a maze, the door must be thick enough to provide shielding equivalent to the wall surrounding the door. For mega-voltage vaults, the door would be very thick and heavy and therefore slow to open and close.

Answer 9

TVL stands for tenth value layer for a specific material and is used to describe thicknesses required for shielding. One tenth-value layer is defined as the amount of shielding material required to reduce the radiation intensity to one tenth of the unshielded value. One TVL equals 3.3 half-value layers.

Answer 10

Boron and polyethylene, as they moderate the fast and intermediate energy neutrons.

Question 11

For what energy should a high-dose rate brachytherapy room using an Ir-192 source be shielded?

Question 12

For a PET CT scanner, what component (PET or CT) requires more consideration for shielding?

Question 13

Is more shielding required in the patient holding area or the actual scanning room for PET CT?

Question 14

What is the dose limit for a radiation area?

Answer 11

Although the average energy for Ir-192 is 380 keV, Ir-192 has a relatively wide energy spectrum that can reach 1.06 MeV.

Answer 12

Fluorine-18 (F-18) is the most common isotope for PET. It has a half-life of 110 minutes. It primarily decays by positron emission, eventually resulting in a photon of energy 511 keV. The X-ray energy for a CT scanner is typically below 140 kVp, so the PET component is the main consideration for shielding.

Answer 13

The holding area requires more shielding because the Fluorine-18 (F-18) is injected into the patient one hour before acquiring the PET/CT. The decay of F-18 occurs regardless of whether or not the PET/CT images are acquired. Since the patient spends considerably more time in the holding area, the holding area requires more shielding than the scanning room.

Answer 14

The dose limit for a radiation area is 0.05 mSv/hr (5 mrem/hr) at 30 cm from the source. An example of a radiation area would be a CT simulator. A sign must be posted to alert individuals.

Question 15

What is the dose limit for a high radiation area?

Question 16

What signage is required outside of a high-dose rate brachytherapy afterloader room?

Answer 15

The dose limit for a high radiation area is 1 mSv/hr (100 mrem/hr) at 30 cm from the source or any surface the radiation penetrates. An example would be a linear accelerator or high dose rate (HDR) vault, and a sign must be posted.

Answer 16

High Radiation Area and Radioactive Material sign.

13

DIAGNOSTIC IMAGING

KEVIN WUNDERLE, NICHOLAS SHKUMAT, AND FRANK DONG

Question 1   13.1 RADIOGRAPHY AND FLUOROSCOPY

Why is there a significant difference in image contrast between a general radiograph and a portal image (or film) of the same patient and same anatomy?

Question 2

What is the general range of kVps used for diagnostic imaging?

Question 3

For all diagnostic X-ray imaging, where does the depth of maximum dose (D_{max}) reside?

Question 4

Assuming no other changes, as the image receptor is moved farther away from the patient, what happens to the anatomy in the image?

Answer 1

The greater contrast in the general radiographic image results from lower energy photons (kilovoltage) having a larger fraction of photoelectric interactions. This is especially apparent when bone is imaged. The photoelectric effect is proportional to $(Z/E)^3$; therefore, high-Z and low-E result in very large absorption, hence increased contrast. In comparison, portal images in radiation therapy use the megavoltage (MV) energy treatment beam. For MV energy photons, Compton scattering is the dominant interaction with tissue. Compton interactions are dependent on electron density, which varies minimally between tissue types.

Answer 2

The typical operational range of kVps for diagnostic imaging is between 60 and 120 kVp. The kVp used for a given exam will depend on the anatomy to be imaged and the desired image quality.

Answer 3

D_{max} resides at the skin surface for diagnostic energy X-ray beams; there is essentially no buildup depth for kilovoltage X-rays.

Answer 4

As the image receptor is moved away from the patient with no other changes in geometry, the anatomy in the image will be magnified. The magnification factor will be equal to the source to image distance/source to object distance (SID/SOD).

Question 5

In an automatic exposure control (AEC) or automatic brightness control (ABC) image acquisition, moving the patient as close to the image receptor as possible will have what effect on patient skin entrance dose?

Question 6

For X-ray-based angiography, what are the two primary factors contributing to blurring of the vessels in the image?

Question 7

What are the patient dose limits for radiographic and/or fluoroscopic procedures?

Question 8

For all modern fluoroscopic units (manufactured after 2006), the cumulative air kinetic energy released per unit mass (kerma) is required to be displayed. Is the cumulative air kerma equivalent to the patient skin dose?

Answer 5

Reducing the distance between the patient and the image receptor for an AEC or ABC image acquisition will reduce the patient skin entrance dose. Dose reduction will be proportional to $(\text{SSD}_{initial}/\text{SSD}_{final})^2$ (inverse square law), where SSD is source to skin distance.

Answer 6

The two primary factors contributing to blurring of vessels in an image are the focal spot size and the location of the anatomy in relation to the image receptor (greater distance results in greater geometric blur).

Answer 7

There are no regulatory limits for patient radiation dose for radiographic or fluoroscopic procedures. However, the Joint Commission does define a sentinel event for fluoroscopic procedures resulting in a cumulative skin dose of 15 Gy, or more, to a single field.

Answer 8

The displayed air kerma on fluoroscopes is an air kerma calculated to a reference plane. The reported air kerma is the sum of all radiation output, in all projections. Therefore, this value does not directly relate to a skin dose since it does not account for the geometric dose distribution. Additionally, the reported air kerma can substantially deviate from the skin dose because it does not account for the accuracy of the ion chamber (which may deviate by ±35%), attenuation factors of the table and pad (which can exceed 30%), tissue back scatter factors, and f-factors based on photon energy.

Question 9

For imaging performed with image intensifier-based fluoroscopes, where in the image field of view should the anatomy of interest be placed?

Question 10

What is the conversion sequence of the image signal, starting with the X-rays exiting the patient and ending with the output phosphor, in an image intensifier?

Question 11

For fluoroscopic imaging, when the field of view (FOV) is changed by increasing the magnification, how is the air kinetic energy released per unit mass (kerma) rate at a fixed location affected?

Question 12

State-of-the-art fluoroscopic systems use dynamic copper (Cu) filtration. What is the purpose of these filters and how do they affect image quality?

Answer 9

All image intensifiers have some geometric distortion that typically increases near the periphery of the image; therefore, the anatomy of interest should be placed in the center of the image.

Answer 10

The X-rays leave the patient and pass through the grid, where some are absorbed. They then reach the input phosphor, where the X-rays are converted to light. Directly behind the input phosphor, the light photons are converted to electrons by the photocathode. The electrons are accelerated across the evacuated tube and strike the output phosphor, converting the electrons back to light.

Answer 11

When the FOV is decreased (by increased magnification) the air kerma rate will increase. For image intensifier-based systems, the increase will be proportional to the square of the ratio of beam areas $(A_2/A_1)^2$. For digital image receptors, generally the air kerma rate increases; however, the increase is not necessarily related to the beam area.

Answer 12

The Cu filters are used to harden the X-ray beam, thereby reducing the skin entrance dose. However, as an X-ray beam is hardened there is a subsequent loss of contrast in the image.

Question 13

Assuming that other factors do not change; does reducing the X-ray field size by collimation reduce the air kerma (kinetic energy released per unit mass) rate, the air-kerma-area-product rate (AKAP) or both?

Question 14

If the air-kerma-area-product rate (AKAP; kerma: kinetic energy released per unit mass) is measured free-in-air 50 cm from an X-ray source and then again at 100 cm from the same X-ray source, how does this measurement change?

Question 15

Which image receptor has the highest potential spatial resolution: an image intensifier, a digital flat panel detector, or traditional film?

Question 1   13.2 MRI

In T2-weighted MRI of the prostate, a tumor is visibly darker than the surrounding normal tissue. Why?

Answer 13

The AKAP rate will be reduced, but the air kerma rate will remain unchanged. Air kerma is normalized to mass (just like dose), so the field size will not affect the air kerma. However, AKAP is the product of the air kerma and the field size, therefore a change in the beam area will have a direct effect.

Answer 14

AKAP is not impacted by the plane of measurement; therefore, the values will be identical. Even though the air kerma decreases by the inverse square law with distance from a radiation source, the area of the beam increases by the same proportion.

Answer 15

The spatial resolution capabilities for film are much greater than for any other current image receptor. The primary benefit of using a digital detector is the ability it offers the operator to adjust the window and level, providing dynamic contrast adjustment.

Answer 1

The T2 relaxation time of the tumor tissue is less than that of the surrounding tissue. This shortened T2 results in greater transverse dephasing yielding decreased signal and a darker appearance in the image.

Question 2

For MRI, what is the requirement regarding the atomic mass number (A)?

Question 3

What effect does increasing the strength of the slice-select gradient have on the image thickness?

Question 4

If MRI is used to scan an anatomic region with a high proportion of fat, what common methods of fat suppression (pulse sequences) are available?

Question 5

How do most contrast agents used in MRI work?

Answer 2

The atomic mass number (A) must be odd (an odd number of either protons or neutrons) for there to be a net magnetic moment of the nucleus, which is required for MRI to function.

Answer 3

For a fixed radio frequency (RF) bandwidth, the image slice thickness will decrease when the slice-select gradient strength is increased. This improves spatial resolution and reduces volume averaging in the slice thickness dimension.

Answer 4

The use of an inversion recovery pulse sequence such as a short tau inversion recovery (STIR) with an appropriate time of inversion (TI), Dixon technique (phase suppression), and chemical shift saturation (spectral suppression) are common techniques that suppress fat signal.

Answer 5

T1 relaxation agents are the primary type of contrast agent used in MRI. These agents speed up the spin-lattice energy transfer (reducing the local T1 relaxation time), thereby increasing the T1 signal.

Question 6

How do contrast agents used in MRI differ from contrast agents used in computed tomography (CT) or other X-ray-based imaging modalities?

Question 7

What is a typical in-plane spatial resolution and an estimate of the highest resolution possible for clinically approved MRI units?

Question 8

What are a few of the benefits of increasing the primary magnetic field strength (B_0) (eg, why use 3T or greater versus 1.5T)?

Question 9

What are a few of the detriments of increasing the primary magnetic field strengths?

Answer 6

Contrast agents used in X-ray-based imaging modalities have a higher atomic number than the surrounding tissue and therefore absorb photons via photoelectric effect, making the contrast agent directly visible in the image. Most MRI contrast agents affect the local T1 relaxation times of the tissue environment in which they are present. This enhances image contrast on a T1-weighted protocol; the contrast agents are not directly visible in the image, but their effects are.

Answer 7

Typical in-plane resolution is similar to that of CT, with a pixel size between 0.5 and 1.0 mm. With a small field of view (FOV) and a high-strength gradient on a surface coil, pixel size can be as small as 0.1 mm.

Answer 8

Assuming all other parameters are unchanged, a larger B_0 provides a greater signal to noise ratio (SNR). If an SNR equivalent to that seen with a lower field strength is acceptable; the image slice thickness can be reduced, which decreases partial volume averaging, or the same slice thickness can be used with a reduced number of signal averages, reducing the acquisition time. A larger B_0 also allows for better discrimination in MR spectroscopy.

Answer 9

T1 relaxation is dependent on the primary magnetic field strength; a higher B_0 requires higher radio frequency (RF) and greater power, which deposits more energy (heat) into the tissue. Higher RF waves result in reduced penetration, which presents image quality issues especially for deep tissue imaging. Many artifacts, such as chemical shift, are exacerbated by increasing B_0.

Question 10

Is there any benefit to performing MR spectroscopy in neuroimaging?

Question 1   **13.3 MAMMOGRAPHY**

Why is a relatively low kVp used in mammography (23–35 kVp) versus the kVp used in other X-ray examinations (abdominal X-ray = 80 kVp; chest X-ray = 120 kVp)?

Question 2

Breasts are compressed during mammographic imaging, typically at 15 to 25 lbs of pressure. Why is this done?

Question 3

What are the factors that allow calcifications to be highly visible at the X-ray energies used in mammographic imaging?

Answer 10

Choline, N-acetylaspartate (NAA), and lactate levels (among others) can be determined, providing valuable clinical information. Higher choline levels have been linked to rapid cellular turnover and tissue growth. Decreases in NAA indicate the potential for necrosis. Lactate levels are linked to the presence of anaerobic conditions and ischemia.

Answer 1

The difference in X-ray attenuation coefficients between normal and abnormal breast tissue is extremely small versus the differences seen with pathologies in other anatomic regions. As subject contrast is inversely proportional to X-ray energy, imaging the patient at a low energy increases the potential for visualizing small tissue dissimilarities.

Answer 2

Compressing the breast increases image uniformity, as the tissue is "spread" across the receptor. This reduces the effective thickness of the breast, increasing effective contrast (healthy tissue is more compressible than abnormal tissue) and reducing X-ray scatter, exposure time, and patient dose. Compression also immobilizes the tissue, minimizing the potential for motion artifacts.

Answer 3

The X-ray attenuation of tissue is dependent on many factors, including physical density, electron density, and atomic number. Calcifications appear highly visible at mammographic energies because of their high effective atomic number ($Z \approx 14$ versus $Z \approx 7$ for breast tissue) and the photoelectric interaction, which is proportional to Z^3.

Question 4

Digital breast tomosynthesis, a new modality recently approved for clinical use, claims to improve which facets of breast imaging?

Question 5

Although analog (screen/film) mammography remains in a small percentage of facilities nationwide, what are the major benefits of upgrading to full-field digital mammography?

Question 6

How do mammographic anti-scatter grids differ from those used in general radiography?

Question 7

What are the advantages and disadvantages of magnification mammographic imaging?

Answer 4

This technique may potentially improve imaging accuracy, improve overall mass conspicuity, and decrease recall rates when compared to digital mammography.

Answer 5

Major advantages include benefits in image storage, archival, and transmission; the ability to manipulate and process images, increased patient throughput; reduced nominal patient dose per acquisition; and elimination of film processing uncertainties and costs. Benefits with regard to patient care include potential improvements in early cancer detection, reduced recall rates, and decreased false-negative biopsy results.

Answer 6

Mammographic grids oscillate to remove the appearance of grid lines. Mammographic grids are also designed with a lower grid ratio and grid frequency (less scatter is removed), and the interspace materials are less attenuating than those used in general radiography.

Answer 7

Magnification mammography improves the effective contrast and resolution when compared to contact imaging. This allows for improved differentiation of spatial distribution/morphology of microcalcifications, and improved visualization of the periphery of masses. Common downsides of magnification imaging are increased exposure times due to the use of a smaller focal spot, as well as increased patient dose per view.

Question 8

The Code of Federal Regulations (CFR) states, "The average glandular dose delivered during a single cranio-caudal view of an FDA-accepted phantom simulating a standard breast shall not exceed 3.0 milligray (mGy) (0.3 rad) per exposure" CFR §21, 900.12(e)(5)(vi). What is the limit for a single clinical breast image?

Question 9

Automatic exposure control (AEC) is used for all routine mammographic acquisitions. Under which area of the breast should the AEC region be positioned?

Question 10

What is the most common class of digital mammography detectors, and what is their defining difference from those used for general radiography?

Question 1   13.4 NUCLEAR IMAGING

What are the benefits of acquiring a CT scan with a single-photon emission CT (SPECT) or PET acquisition?

Answer 8

There is no dose limit on the acquisition of patient images. The FDA limit only applies to the dose deliver to an approved phantom of specific composition. The mean glandular dose delivered per view of an average breast (4.2 cm compressed) is approximately 1 mGy (digital mammography).

Answer 9

The AEC is ideally positioned under the most attenuating (densest and thickest) area of the patient's breast. This is to ensure adequate penetration and appropriate noise characteristics for the most demanding anatomic region.

Answer 10

Most mammographic digital detectors are full-field, active-matrix, thin-film transistor devices. They are integrated directly into the mammography stand and are categorized as either direct-detection [using an amorphous-selenium (a-Se) photoconductor] or indirect-detection (using a scintillator as an intermediary step in the detection process) devices. The characteristic difference between mammographic and radiographic detectors is the physical size of the detector element (del). Mammographic del typically ranges from 0.050 to 0.1 mm, where radiographic del is upward of 0.2 mm.

Answer 1

A hardware-registered CT allows for anatomic discrimination of the functional nuclear medicine examination, which leads to improved localization of lesions that present with increased radiotracer uptake. The second benefit is that CT can be used to correct nuclear medicine images for patient attenuation. CT correction provides low-noise correction factors with a short scan time and without bias from the injected isotope.

Question 2

What is the most commonly used radiopharmaceutical in PET?

Question 3

How would you describe the decay scheme for F-18?

Question 4

What is the standardized uptake value (SUV)?

Question 5

What are common sources of variability with PET standardized uptake value (SUV)?

Answer 2

Fluorodeoxyglucose (FDG) using F-18. A glucose analog, FDG is absorbed by high-glucose-using areas of the body, including the brain, heart, and cancer cells. Because of FDGs construction, once this radiopharmaceutical has been absorbed within a cell, it cannot be further metabolized and thus remains within the cell during the process of radioactive decay. This makes FDG a strong indicator of body glucose distribution.

Answer 3

In 97% of cases, F-18 decays through positron emission; a proton is transformed into a neutron, and emits a positron and neutrino. The positron has a maximum energy of 0.633 MeV, with the remaining energy transferred to the neutrino.

Positron Decay: $^{18}_{9}F \rightarrow {}^{18}_{8}O + {}^{0}_{+1}\beta e + v$

In the remaining 3% of cases, F-18 decays through electron capture.

Answer 4

SUV is a simplified quantitative metric used in PET imaging. This value represents the radioisotope uptake within a region of interest measured at a time interval after tracer administration and normalized to the injected dose and to a factor that accounts for the body activity distribution. Typically normalized to patient weight, SUV may also be modified to account for lean body mass, body surface area, and plasma glucose concentration.

Answer 5

Quantitative PET performance can be affected by three general forms of variability: biological variability, procedural variability, and variability associated with the system. Biological sources include patient compliance issues (eg, fasting, anxiety) and physiological variability (eg, blood glucose level). Procedural sources include scan parameters, such as the time between injection and imaging, scan duration, 2 dimensional / 3 dimensional (2D/3D) acquisition, and patient motion issues. System sources of variability include calibration procedures and protocols performed by the medical physicist, quality assurance, inherent system characteristics, and image processing.

Question 6

What is the most commonly used radioisotope in nuclear medicine imaging?

Question 7

Yttrium-90 (Y-90) can be used for targeted radionuclide therapy. How is its radiotracer biodistribution imaged after the administration of a therapeutic dose?

Question 8

Collimators are always used during gamma camera imaging. What effect does increasing the parallel hole collimator-to-object distance have on sensitivity, spatial resolution, and image magnification?

Question 9

What is the approximate detection efficiency and energy resolution of 140.5 keV (Tc-99m) photons in a gamma camera (with 10-mm-thick NaI(Tl)).

Answer 6

Technetium-99m (Tc-99m). This radioisotope is an artificially produced, metastable isotope of technetium-99 that decays through isomeric transition. Tc-99m is valuable in nuclear medicine because of its physical half-life of 6.01 hours (>90% decay within 24 hours), 140.5 keV gamma rays (minimal patient attenuation, efficient detection in gamma cameras), and short biological half-life. Tc-99m is also easily bound to various biologically active substances.

Answer 7

Y-90 is a primary beta-particle emitter with a 0.01% gamma emission at 1.7 MeV. As photons of that energy are not conducive or appropriate for gamma camera or single-photon emission CT (SPECT) imaging, one solution is to image the bremsstrahlung photons generated through the interaction of the beta emissions with nuclei within the patient.

Answer 8

With a parallel hole collimator, as the patient moves farther from the camera, the spatial resolution decreases, and the sensitivity decreases very slightly (approximately constant). Image magnification remains constant. These characteristics differ when converging, diverging, or pinhole collimators are used.

Answer 9

The detection efficiency approaches 85% at 140 keV, with a corresponding energy resolution of approximately 10%.

Question 10

What are the three main causes of quantitative error in PET coincident event detection?

Question 11

PET imaging can be acquired in 2D or 3D mode. What are the advantages and disadvantages of 3D imaging?

Question 12

"Time-of-flight" (TOF) is a new method of PET data acquisition (TOF-PET). What is the primary advantage of TOF-PET over a non-TOF system?

Question 1   13.5 CT

Why are Hounsfield units (HU) for the same biologic tissue different when images are acquired on two different CT scanners? (Assume the same scanning techniques, the same kVp and mA values, and similar reconstruction kernels are used.)

Answer 10

The primary causes of quantitative error in event detection are lost events due to attenuation or photons not incident on the detector, scattered coincident events, and random coincident events. No line of response (LOR) is created during lost events, whereas scattered and random events create false LOR.

Answer 11

3D PET offers a considerable increase in imaging sensitivity, up to a factor of 5. This can allow for an image with improved noise characteristics or a significantly reduced acquisition time. The primary downside is an increased proportion of scattered and random events. Modern scanners can acquire in 2D and 3D modes or exclusively in 3D modes.

Answer 12

TOF-PET allows for the improved localization of coincident events. This results in an improvement in the overall signal to noise ratio (SNR). This gain can be used in the form of improved image quality or reduced acquisition time.

Answer 1

Different CT scanners, especially from two different CT vendors, may have different X-ray spectra (photon energy distribution); therefore, the attenuation, even for the same tissue-equivalent material, may be different on two different scanners. HU is proportional to the linear attenuation coefficient; therefore, the HU values may be different. In fact, for a well-calibrated CT scanner, only two materials, water and air, have "defined" HU values (0 HU ± 7 HU and −1,000 HU ± 5 HU, respectively), and these values are independent of the CT manufacturer.

Question 2

A patient undergoes a three-phase liver CT study. For the venous phase, will the average CT number (Hounsfield units [HU]) around the portal vein be different under 100 kVp than at 120 kVp? If so, which kVp scan will have a higher CT number?

Question 3

Typically, liver lesions have very low contrast compared to the surrounding liver parenchyma. Assuming the lesions are >5 mm, which change would you select first to increase the lesion detectability? Which one will you select as the last measure to increase the lesion detectability? (a) Increase tube current from 200 to 400 mA, (b) increase slice thickness from 2.5 to 5 mm, or (c) use a smooth reconstruction kernel.

Question 4

What is a 4DCT?

Question 5

What are the differences in imaging dose and quality of a 4D compared to 3DCT?

Answer 2

For iodine contrast, the CT number will be enhanced more under 100 kVp than at 120 kVp, because the k-edge of iodine is closer to the effective photon energy of 100 kVp than to that of 120 kVp; therefore, the attenuation is higher for a 100-kVp X-ray beam when it passes the portal vein filled with iodine contrast, resulting in a higher average CT number (or HU).

Answer 3

It is preferable to start with (c) to see whether the detectability is sufficient; (b) is the next best option to increase detectability, but at the cost of lower spatial resolution or partial volume artifacts. The least desirable option is (a) because of increased dose to the patient. Options (b) and (c) are both reconstruction parameters and therefore do not affect the dose delivered to the patient. Option (a) will increase the dose to the patient by approximately two times.

Answer 4

A 4DCT comprises 3DCTs of the patient at different phases of the breathing cycle, typically divided into 8 or 10 phases. The breathing cycle signal is measured by a spirometer, strain gauge belt, or infra-red reflective block and camera. The measured signal is then sampled either according to the breathing cycle time or amplitude into the multiple phases. The 4DCT can be viewed in cine mode to observe the motion.

Answer 5

4DCTs clearly require a larger imaging dose, in order to image the same volume multiple times. Some of this increase in dose can be mitigated by reducing the quality of the 4DCT image, so that a 4DCT may not be 10 times greater in dose. The 4DCT has the advantage of reduced motion artifacts over a 3DCT.

Question 6

In helical 4DCT acquisition for the stereotactic radiosurgery of lung cancer, the pitch factor has to be small enough to prevent image artifacts. Which of the following factors may affect the selection of the pitch factor: (a) the duration of one breath cycle, (b) the patient size, (c) the detector collimation, or (d) the maximum tube current?

Question 7

In a 4DCT how are maximum intensity projection (MIP) and average scans produced, and what are their uses?

Question 8

How does a lung tumor appear in an average versus a maximum intensity projection (MIP) scan?

Question 9

What is the cause of the image artifact in the following image (see arrow in image)?

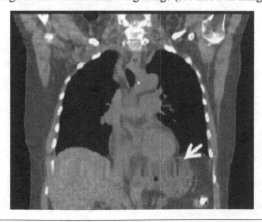

Answer 6

In 4DCT acquisition, the data sufficient condition (DSC) requires the data to be acquired within one breath hold; therefore, (a) is the correct answer.

Answer 7

The information contained in a 4DCT can be condensed into a single synthetic 3DCT using methods, such as MIP or average intensity projection (AIP). A MIP takes the maximum intensity of a given voxel in all phases of the 4DCT and assigns this as the intensity in the new 3DCT. Similarly, the AIP uses the average intensity of the voxel in the 4DCT. A minimum intensity projection is also available. Further, these projections can be determined over just a subset of the 4DCT phases. For example, if you plan to gate and treat just in the 80% to 100% phase, you would use just those images to create your MIP for planning.

Answer 8

An average scan will smear the location of the tumor. It will look similar but not the same as a free breathing 3DCT. On a free breathing CT, the tumor's center of the mass may shift, depending on the phase of the breathing at the acquisition. The tumor in the MIP scan will appear much larger, comprising the entire range of motion of the tumor. Because of the slow acquisition time, the center of the mass of the tumor observed in a cone beam CT (acquired for imaging verification) is more consistent with the center of the mass of the tumor in the average intensity projection (AIP) CT.

Answer 9

The artifact is caused by undersampling of prolonged irregular breathing pattern.

Pan T, Sun X, Luo D. Improvement of the cine-CT-based 4DCT imaging. *Med Phys*. 2007;34:4499

Question 10
Which of the following is the largest potential contributor to geometric inaccuracy of CT imaging: tube focal spot size, collimator, detector cell size, or location of the isocenter?

Question 11
What scanner parameters (may be more than one) affect the spatial resolution of CT imaging: (a) focal spot size, (b) CT tube current, (c) helical pitch, or (d) reconstruction kernel (algorithm)?

Question 12
Iodinated intravenous contrast is the most frequently used contrast agent in CT imaging. How does this agent work?

Question 13
Which of the CT imaging tasks will benefit from the use of iodinated intravenous contrast?

Answer 10

In CT, the location of the isocenter used in the image reconstruction should match the physical location of the isocenter. Any deviation from the assumed isocenter to the physical isocenter will cause geometric distortion and thus reduce accuracy; therefore, location of the isocenter is the largest contributor.

Answer 11

(a) and (d) are the best answers. In general, a CT scanner has two focal spot sizes. The small focal spot is used for studies that require high resolution, such as the inner ear canal, whereas the large focal spot is used mainly for chest imaging and spinal and abdominal imaging, which do not require superior spatial resolution. The reconstruction kernel (sometimes called the reconstruction algorithm) can shape the frequency response of the CT projection data during the filtered back-projection reconstruction, either to boost or reduce the spatial resolution. In CT, the spatial resolution boost from the reconstruction kernel is at the cost of image noise (ie, high spatial resolution kernel brings higher image noise).

Answer 12

Iodinated contrast works by increasing the number of photons attenuated within the vessels. Iodine's k-edge is slightly lower than the effective photon energy from a CT X-ray beam; therefore, attenuation is much higher for the vessel filled with iodine contrast, providing image contrast.

Answer 13

Iodinated contrast requires blood flow. Solid lesions have enough blood supply to appear as areas of high intensity on the image, but cystic lesions do not have a blood supply; therefore, cystic lesions will appear as areas of low intensity (water-like) on contrast images. Imaging of lung nodules, kidney stones, or bone fractures would not be improved.

Question 14

In CT, metal implants can cause severe image artifacts shown as bright or dark streaks/bands surrounding the metal object. What is the main cause of these artifacts?

Question 15

Scatter radiation to the CT detector is the main contributor to degraded CT image quality. Scatter radiation is primarily generated within the patient and secondarily from the hardware itself (such as from the second tube in a dual-source scanner). What is the major effect of scatter radiation on the CT image?

Question 16

The volume CT dose index (CTDIvol) can be determined using two different right cylindrical acrylic phantoms: a 16-cm diameter phantom for pediatric and head protocols and a 32-cm diameter phantom for adult body protocols. For measurements made in each phantom, with identical scan parameters, which will have a greater CTDIvol?

Question 1   13.6 ULTRASOUND

Which is the primary factor determining the axial resolution of B-mode (brightness mode) imaging?

Answer 14

The main cause of metal artifacts is a paucity of photons penetrating the metal object. Secondarily, those photons that do penetrate the object to form the image are heavily filtered and will cause strong beam hardening artifacts.

Answer 15

The main effect is CT number shift. If the detector receives excessive radiation, the total signal it generates increases, decreasing the apparent attenuation from the patient, and reducing the CT number.

Answer 16

CTDIvol determined from measurements in the 16-cm CTDI phantom will be greater than that from the 32-cm phantom given identical scan parameters (less attenuating material). If the CTDIvol is determined using the wrong phantom, the reported value will be overestimated if the 16-cm phantom was used for an adult body protocol or underestimated if the 32-cm phantom was used for a pediatric or head protocol.

Answer 1

The spatial pulse length is the primary factor. As rule of thumb, the axial resolution = 1/2 × (spatial pulse length). The pulse amplitude will affect the B-mode signal strength. The center frequency will affect the attenuation of the signal. The width of the transducer element may affect the center frequency of the pulse.

Question 2

In ultrasound, what will provide the best benefit to the lateral resolution in the image (the lateral direction is perpendicular to the pulse transmitting direction)?

Question 3

In ultrasound, transmit or receive gain is measured in the unit of decibels (dB). If the receive gain is 3 dB, what is the amplification factor for the output power versus the input power?

Question 4

One of the fundamental physics principles governing ultrasound image quality is the attenuation coefficient of the pulse-echo signal. The attenuation coefficient is linearly proportional to the center frequency. For most soft tissues, what is this linear attenuation coefficient?

Question 5

Doppler color flow imaging and power Doppler imaging both use color-coded pixel values to indicate blood flow information. What is the major difference between these two modes?

Answer 2

Placing the focal zone or multiple focal zones around the region of interest. In ultrasound, the best lateral resolution can be found at the center of the focal zone. All commercial ultrasound scanners should have multiple focal zones available, which will provide a wide range of depth with good spatial resolution. The tradeoff to these multiple focal zones is a slow frame rate.

Answer 3

dB is log scale = $10 \times \log A$, where A is the amplification factor. Since $3\ dB = 10 \times \log 2$, 3 dB means the output power is two times the input power.

Answer 4

For most soft tissues, the linear attenuation coefficient is 0.5 dB/cm/MHz (ie, the attenuation is 3 dB/cm if the center frequency is 6 MHz, or the signal will decrease by half of its original strength for each centimeter of soft tissue traveled for a 6-MHz pulse).

Answer 5

Color flow imaging can detect the flow direction, but power Doppler cannot. Power Doppler uses only the amplitude of the flow, not the phase; therefore, this technique is less sensitive to aliasing artifacts. However, power Doppler is more sensitive to flow information in small vessels.

Question 6

How would lung, bone, air cavity, and bladder affect ultrasound shadowing artifact?

Question 7

Reverberation artifacts in ultrasound are due to multiple reflections between a structure and the transducer or multiple reflections within a structure itself. Reverberations degrade image quality and may overlay lesions, potentially leading to misdiagnosis. Is there any simple way to reduce reverberation artifacts?

Question 8

How does 3D ultrasound work?

Question 9

What is the frequency of the waves used in medical ultrasound devices? What is the speed of ultrasound in tissue?

Answer 6

Ultrasound shadowing artifacts are due to reduced echo intensity behind highly attenuating objects, such as an air cavity or a stone. The bladder is the least attenuating organ, it is unlikely to generate shadowing artifacts.

Answer 7

A simple method to reduce reverberations is to angle the probe slightly to avoid direct incidence onto a flat surface.

Answer 8

Standard ultrasound scanning produces 2D images. 2D images at multiple depths may be taken. To get a true 3D image, sound waves are sent at different angles, instead of from one main direction in 2D ultrasound. Their echoes are then collected and processed in a similar way to CT reconstruction of transmitted X-rays.

Answer 9

Medical ultrasound devices typically operate in the 1 to 20 MHz range. Typically speed of ultrasound in tissue is 1,540 ms^{-1}

Question 10

How is ultrasound frequency related to wavelength, and how does this affect resolution?

Question 11

Why does native tissue harmonic imaging have a relatively large imaging depth even though it uses higher frequency echo signals to form images (second harmonic, ie, two times fundamental frequency)?

Answer 10

The wavelength is inversely proportional to frequency. Hence, higher frequency waves have a shorter wavelength, while lower frequency waves have a longer wavelength. A high-frequency wave will give better axial resolution, but it will be attenuated more and will not penetrate as deep as a low-frequency wave. On the other hand, a low-frequency wave will penetrate deeper at the expense of resolution.

Answer 11

Native tissue harmonic is formed from the fundamental frequency sound waves traveling to depth or during the harmonic echoed return to the transducer. The harmonic component of the sound waves travels only one way, not both ways like the fundamental frequency sound wave component. Increased attenuation of the higher harmonic components only occurs during the portion of the trip in which they are present, reducing their attenuation. Therefore, native tissue harmonic imaging can still maintain significant imaging depth.

14

IMAGE GUIDANCE

ERIC TISCHLER AND LAMA MUHIEDDINE MOSSOLLY

Question 1

What is IGRT and why is it used?

Question 2

What is the difference between accuracy and precision?

Question 3

What are some examples of both inter-fraction and intra-fraction variables that cause uncertainty in treatment targeting during radiation therapy?

Question 4

What are the different systems used for image-guided radiation therapy (IGRT)?

Answer 1

IGRT: image-guided radiation therapy. It is used to ensure that the treatment target is localized and aligned to the radiation beams as in the images that are used to plan the treatment before delivering radiation therapy.

Answer 2

Accuracy is how close the measured value is to the true value. Precision is how close the measured values are to each other. It is possible to be precise without being accurate, and accurate without being precise. The aim of image-guided radiation therapy (IGRT) is accuracy.

Answer 3

Patient positioning/setup errors, weight loss, change in volumes, and bladder/rectum filling are a few examples of changes that can occur from fraction to fraction (inter-fraction). Patient movement during treatment, breathing, gas movement in the bowels, and cardiac motion are a few factors that can lead to uncertainty during treatment (intra-fraction).

Answer 4

Electronic portal imaging device (EPID), two-dimensional kilovoltage imaging pair, stereoscopic kilovoltage images, megavoltage cone beam (MVCT), kilovoltage cone beam (kVCT), CT-on-rails (in-room diagnostic quality CT scan), optical tracking, in-room magnetic resonance imaging, ultrasound (US), electromagnetic transponders.

Question 5
What is the process of image-guided radiation therapy (IGRT)?

Question 6
How does an electronic portal imaging device (EPID) work?

Question 7
What is cone beam imaging and how is it different from a regular CT?

Question 8
What are the disadvantages and advantages of megavoltage computed tomography (MVCT) in radiation therapy?

Answer 5

The IGRT process is similar among the different methods. The patient is first positioned on the treatment table in the same way they were simulated, using the room laser to align the machine isocenter with the marked isocenter on the patient body. Images of the patient are acquired using one of the listed IGRT systems. The acquired IGRT images are registered with the reference images, focusing on the specified anatomy. The registration is used to determine the initial patient offset required to align the target with the planned treatment beams. The repositioning software will display the offset as shifts for the treatment couch to align the patient in the same position as planned.

Answer 6

The incoming X-rays interact with the scintillation screen that converts them into optical wavelength photons. The optical photons are detected by the amorphous silicon photodiodes, which then are converted into an electronic signal and image.

Answer 7

Cone beam imaging uses a cone-shaped X-ray beam that transmits onto a detector creating a complete volume image with one rotation. A regular CT images the patient with a narrow collimation creating a fan shaped X-ray beam. The narrow collimated beam images a thin "slice" of the patient. Therefore, while the fan beam rotates around the patient, the couch must slowly move along the longitudinal direction, resulting in a helical (spiral motion) of the X-ray beam, to fully image the patient.

Answer 8

Disadvantages: MVCT uses mega voltage energies where the Compton scattering dominates, so soft tissue is harder to visualize than in kV images where the photoelectric effect dominates. To obtain a good quality image you may need to increase the imaging dose, which causes an increase in radiation exposure to patients. Bony anatomy and tissue with low density (such as air cavity or lung) are visible.

Advantages: The artifacts from large implanted metals are minimized which makes the MV images easier to visualize the anatomy near metal implants than in kV images. The imaging beam and treatment beam also share the same isocenter, preventing potential mis-concordance between the imaging center and treatment center. Linear accelerator (linac)-based kV cone beam computed tomography (CBCT), however, requires a separate kV source that is placed orthogonal to the treatment beam with a discordance between the imaging and treatment center that could cause an offset between imaging and treatment.

Question 9
What are the advantages of using CT-on-rails?

Question 10
What is infrared optical tracking and how is it used?

Question 11
What is the Calypso 4D Localization system and how does it work?

Question 12
How is the optical tracking system different from that of the electromagnetic transponder system?

Answer 9

CT-on-rails is a diagnostic quality CT located in the same vault as the linear accelerator (linac). It has the same quality images as the planning CT. This increases the accuracy of registering the treatment verification and planning images. The CT images taken with CT-on-rails can also be used for adaptive replanning purpose as they have accurate electron density information.

Answer 10

Optical tracking uses passive or active infrared markers that are detected by a camera. These markers are placed on the surface of the patient and are useful to detect both the patient position relative to the plan and whether the patient moves during treatment. A calibration method associates the camera's coordinates with that of the isocenter of the treatment machine.

Answer 11

The Calypso system has been referred to as a global positioning satellite (GPS) for the body, and is a common form of image-guided radiation therapy (IGRT) used for prostate patients receiving external beam therapy. Tiny transponder beacons (8.5 mm long, 1.85 mm diameter) are implanted into the prostate during an outpatient procedure. The locations of these transponders infer the prostate position and rotation. The Calypso tracking system communicates with these transponders via radio waves. Calypso systems can track the prostate position and motion in nearly real time (20 times a second).

During radiation delivery, users can set a prostate position threshold above which the radiation beam will be stopped. Using the Calypso system, high radiation doses can be confidently delivered to the target with tighter margins, sparing normal tissue, and reducing unwanted side effects.

www.varian.com/oncology/products/real-time-tracking/calypso-extracranial-tracking?cat=overview

Answer 12

The optical tracking markers are placed on the surface of the patient's body. The electromagnetic transponders are typically implanted into an organ (such as the prostate). This will provide a real time tracking method of the organ. The transponders are activated by radiofrequency waves. Both tracking methods are considered a form of image-guided radiation therapy (IGRT) because they are used for the same purpose of aligning the target with the planned treatment beams.

Question 13

What are the benefits and disadvantages of the ultrasound (US) for image-guided radiation therapy (IGRT)?

Question 14

What is a common imaging modality used for guidance during radioactive prostate seed implants? Briefly explain how it is used.

Question 15

Discuss the ultrasound (US) for external beam therapy.

Question 16

Would megavoltage cone beam computed tomography (MV CBCT) be a good choice for imaging the prostate during image-guided radiation therapy (IGRT)?

Answer 13

US uses sound waves that are reflected back to the transducer and converts the signal to an image. The US is best used for localization of the prostate and the tumor cavity of the breast, because their locations permit for easy access of the US probe. US is noninvasive and does not produce ionizing radiation. It can be used daily to correct for motion and setup error. The disadvantage of using US is that it is operator dependent. Results may vary depending on how the operator applies the pressure to the probe.

Answer 14

Real-time ultrasound (US) imaging is frequently used during the prostate seed implantation procedure. A trans-rectal US probe is used to capture a series of static images for planning purposes. It is also used to visualize the prostate, surrounding tissue, seeds, and needles during the actual implantation.

Answer 15

In external beam, ultrasound provides soft tissue visualization for the prostate and breast cavity. During the simulation phase, US images can be taken and fused with planning CT images to provide better visualization of the target and surrounding structures. During treatment, US images allow target structures to be aligned using shape, size, and position of anatomy. Ultrasound is advantageous as an imaging method using nonionizing radiation.

Answer 16

For visualizing the actual prostate gland, it would be a poor choice since the MV beam suffers from poor soft-tissue contrast. However, MV CBCT is a common form of IGRT for prostate patients when used in conjunction with fiducials implanted into the gland. The fiducials are highly visible on the MV CBCT and can be used to align it to the reference image.

Question 17

In terms of dose added to the patient's treatment, arrange the following imaging modalities from least to greatest: megavoltage cone beam computed tomography (MV CBCT), planar kV, ultrasound (US), kilovoltage cone beam computed tomography (kV CBCT)

Question 18

What is the difference between random and systematic errors and how do they affect the dose distribution around the clinical tumor volume (CTV)?

Question 19

Define gross tumor volume (GTV), clinical tumor volume (CTV), internal target volume (ITV), and planning target volume (PTV). What effect does image-guided radiation therapy (IGRT) have on these?

Question 20

What is the van Herk formulation for margins?

Answer 17

US (zero dose), planar kV, kV CBCT, MV CBCT.

Answer 18

Random errors are unpredictable and can vary in magnitude and direction from fraction to fraction. This type of error leads to a blurring of the dose distribution around the CTV over the course of treatment. Systematic errors are deviations that occur during each fraction over the entire course of therapy. The deviation is in a similar size and direction and can lead to a shift in the dose distribution away from the CTV.

Answer 19

GTV is the gross, demonstrable extent of the tumor. CTV is the GTV plus additional volume to account for microscopic tumor spread. The ITV is a margin added to the CTV to account for internal physiological movements and position of the CTV during therapy. Finally, the PTV is the volume that includes the CTV and ITV, with an extra margin to account for patient movement, inaccuracies in beam and patient setup, and any other uncertainties. The use of IGRT may lead to a reduction in the margin between the CTV and PTV.

ICRU, Prescribing, Recording and Reporting Photon Beam Therapy Reports 50 & 62, 1993, 1999

Answer 20

For 90% of the patient population, the clinical tumor volume (CTV) would receive 95% of the prescription dose cumulatively in conventional radiation therapy by using a planning target volume (PTV) margin = $2.5 \times$ standard deviation (SD) of the systematic errors + $0.7 \times$ SD of the random errors. Errors arise from organ delineation, motion, and setup.

van Herk M, Remeijer P, Rasch C, Lebesque JV. The probability of correct target dosage: dose-population histograms for deriving treatment margins in radiation therapy. *IJROBP*. 2000;47:1121-1135

Question 21

What are some advantages and disadvantages of using magnetic resonance (MR) for image-guided radiation therapy (IGRT)?

Question 22

Discuss the double-exposure technique that is commonly used for portal imaging.

Question 23

Describe a BB tray and its purpose?

Question 24

Give a brief description of the ExacTrac system.

Answer 21

Advantages: Excellent soft tissue visualization, no radiation dose, and real-time tumor tracking
Disadvantages: Variation in magnetic field can cause geometric distortion of patient images. The magnetic field can also interfere with dose distribution and the function of linear accelerator if no special shielding for the magnetic field is applied.

Answer 22

Portal imaging is used to verify patient position and proper beam shape and size. An exposure is taken with the shaped treatment field to record the treatment portal. Another exposure is taken with an open field to image the surrounding anatomy, allowing easy visualization of how the treatment field relates to this surrounding anatomy. The two exposures are superimposed on the same image.

Answer 23

A BB tray, also known as a graticule or reticle, is a calibrated device with embedded radiographic markers arranged in a cross-like pattern. It is inserted into the tray slot on the linear accelerator. When a portal image is taken, the markers are visible on the image defining the isocenter, x- and y-axes, and scale. This device is mainly used, where the association of the beam isocenter and portal film is not known. Most new machines use a digital graticule where the machine isocenter relative to the electronic portal imager is defined and known.

Answer 24

ExacTrac is a closed loop image-guided radiation therapy (IGRT) system manufactured by Brainlab. ExacTrac uses two stereoscopic X-ray units recessed into the floor on opposite sides of the treatment table and two flat-panel detectors mounted to the ceiling. Patient positioning and movement can be monitored throughout the entire treatment with the integrated optical tracking system and stereoscopic X-rays can be acquired on demand to visualize internal anatomy.

www.brainlab.com/en/radiosurgery-products/exactrac/

Question 25

What are bowtie filters? Describe two types commonly used during cone beam computed tomography (CBCT).

Question 26

What are the advantages of using bowtie filters when performing cone beam computed tomography (CBCT) scans?

Question 27

What energy is typically used for kilovoltage cone beam computed tomography (kV CBCT)?

Question 28

Describe the In-Line kView imaging system that is used by the Siemens Artiste linear accelerator (linac).

Answer 25

Bowtie filters are beam shaping devices for imaging X-rays that can improve the quality of CBCT scans. The half-fan and full-fan bowtie filters are the two common filters. A full-fan bowtie filter's profile is thicker on both sides and thinner in the middle, resembling a bowtie (hence, the name). The thicker ends attenuate the beam more than the central area of the filter. This is usually used for CBCT head scans. A half-fan filter is thicker on one side and thinner on the other. The half-fan mode is used for body scans, where the detector is shifted laterally to increase the imaging axial field-of-view.

Answer 26

Image quality is improved because cupping artifacts induced by X-ray scatter is decreased, and patient skin dose is reduced. Also, higher kVp energy X-rays can be used without saturating the detector, and there is reduced charge trapping in the detector.

Answer 27

Common settings are in the 100 to 125 kVp range for machines equipped with kilovoltage X-ray tubes.

Answer 28

For the Siemens Artiste linac, In-Line kView imaging uses a new MV beam that is produced through a carbon target without the flattening filter. This new imaging beam shifts the energy spectrum closer to the kV range and contains more low-energy X-rays, thus improving soft-tissue contrast when compared to a regular megavoltage cone beam computed tomography (MV CBCT) with the same dose. In-Line means that the imaging center is aligned with the iso-center of the treatment beam as is standard for MV CBCT.

www.healthcare.siemens.com/radiation-oncology/upgrades-and-options-for-your-linac/diagnosis-and-follow-up/cone-beam-ct-imaging-with-in-line-kview

Question 29

Cone beam computed tomography (CBCT) can be acquired by rotating the gantry in a full or half arc. What are the advantages of using a half arc, and are there any disadvantages?

Question 30

Discuss some differences between kV and MV dose deposition in the body.

Question 31

How does beam hardening affect cone beam computed tomography (CBCT)?

Question 32

How is CT-on-rails used in image guidance?

Answer 29

A half arc results in a faster scan, quicker reconstruction, and less dose to the patient. Also, critical surface structures can avoid irradiation, such as the lens of the eye. The trade-off is that images may be of lower quality, have greater noise and suffer from artifacts.

Answer 30

The depth of maximum dose (d_{max}) for typical kV imaging is essentially at the surface, therefore the skin receives a higher dose than MV imaging. Due to the photoelectric effect, bone will also receive a higher dose in kV imaging than in MV imaging. Photons in the kV range are rapidly attenuated as depth in the body increases, as opposed to the photons in the MV range, which is characterized by a buildup, a maximum, and a much slower fall off.

Answer 31

When a polyenergetic X-ray beam passes through an object, lower energy photons are absorbed faster than higher energy photons. The mean energy of the beam increases, and it becomes "harder." This can lead to artifacts in the CBCT.

Answer 32

First, the patient's external marks are aligned to the linear accelerator lasers. BBs are then placed on those marks. The patient is then rotated 180° using the column rotation toward the CT scanner and the CT is acquired. Since the isocenter of the linear accelerator and the acquisition center of CT are not associated, the isocenter coordinates from the two systems are manually associated by using the BBs on the CT image. After imaging registration, the difference between the set isocenter coordinates (BBs) and the reference planning isocenter coordinates is then calculated and displayed. This offset is manually applied after the patient is rotated back 180° and realigned to the linear accelerator lasers.

Question 33

What are some of the registration methods used in image guidance?

Question 34

Describe the four-dimensional cone beam CT (4DCBCT)?

Question 35

What are the disadvantages of four-dimensional cone beam CT (4DCBCT)?

Question 36

Describe the Varian Real-Time Position Management (RPM) System used in radiation therapy?

Answer 33

The methods used for image registration are the mutual information or normalized mutual information, visual alignment, landmarks, and surface matching.

Answer 34

The 4DCBCT is a technique used for image guidance of patients undergoing treatments of a moving target. The 4DCBCT provides a volumetric visualization of the tumor motion at the time of treatment.

Answer 35

4DCBCT requires a longer acquisition time, more imaging dose, and results in poorer imaging quality.

Answer 36

RPM is a noninvasive and real-time tracking system used to measure the chest motion of a patient, which can be linked with the motion of a targeted tumor. It is best used for managing tumor motion in thoracic region and upper abdomen.

apps.varian.com/euen/oncology/radiation_oncology/clinac/rpm_respiratory_gating.html

Question 37
How does Real-Time Position Management (RPM) work?

Question 38
What are the two main ways to divide the breathing cycle?

Question 39
What is the six degrees of freedom (6DoF) couch?

Question 40
What is the typical range of radiation dose given by a kilovoltage cone beam computed tomography (kV CBCT), megavoltage cone beam computed tomography (MV CBCT), and CT-on-rails?

Answer 37

An RPM system uses an infrared camera and reflective block placed on the patient to measure the respiratory cycle based on the movement of the chest. The measured respiratory cycle is recorded as a waveform. The physician uses this waveform to determine the gating thresholds for planning CT acquisition and gated treatment. During gated treatment, the beam will be automatically on if the breathing cycle is above the threshold and off if the breathing cycle is below the thresholds.

apps.varian.com/euen/oncology/radiation_oncology/clinac/rpm_respiratory_gating.html

Answer 38

The two types of breathing cycle binning (dividing the cycle into segments) are phase-binning and amplitude-binning. The phase is defined by selecting time points during the breathing cycle. The amplitude is defined by assigning thresholds in the breathing cycle.

apps.varian.com/euen/oncology/radiation_oncology/clinac/rpm_respiratory_gating.html

Answer 39

The 6DoF couch refers to the movement of the couch in three-dimensional space. The couch moves in the translational directions (superior/inferior, left/right, and up/down) and in the rotational directions (pitch, yaw, and roll).

Answer 40

The radiation dose from any of the in-room CTs varies with the technique used and what body part is imaged. The radiation dose given ranges from 10 to 50 mGy per scan, with CT-on-rails and kV CBCT giving lower doses than MV CBCT.

Question 41

What methods could be applied to reduce the radiation dose to the patient when using the different types of CT used in image guidance?

Question 42

What are fiducial markers and how are they used for image-guided radiation therapy (IGRT) prostate treatments?

Question 43

How are fiducial markers placed in the prostate gland?

Question 44

What other areas use fiducial markers?

Answer 41

Radiation dose can be reduced by adjusting the image acquisition technique used (kVp, mAs, MUs); by minimizing the collimation/jaws to include just the body part of interest, and the use of appropriate filters.

Answer 42

The prostate is difficult to visualize using the onboard X-ray imaging of a linear accelerator. Small fiducial markers made of gold, or other materials can be implanted into the prostate before the course of therapy. Once therapy begins, these markers are highly visible on pretreatment verification images. Their positions are compared to the reference images, and shifts are determined to ensure the prostate is in the correct treatment position.

Answer 43

During a transrectal ultrasound (US), a needle passes through the probe and inserts three markers into the prostate; at the apex, middle, and base of the prostate. This procedure is typically done in an urologist's office.

Answer 44

Fiducial markers are not limited to the prostate and can be used for other treatment targets for which the onboard imaging contrast is insufficient to localize the target. The markers can be deliberately added, or may be surgery related such as stents (pancreas) or clips (eg, breast lumpectomy).

Question 45

What is the Calypso Surface Beacon transponder system?

Question 46

How is imaging performed by a TomoTherapy machine?

Question 47

Is the megavoltage computed tomography (MVCT) on a TomoTherapy unit acceptable for daily use? What is the typical dose given during imaging?

Question 48

What is one difference between megavoltage cone beam computed tomography (MV CBCT) imaging on a conventional linear accelerator versus megavoltage computed tomography (MVCT) on a TomoTherapy unit?

Answer 45

The Surface Beacon by Calypso is similar to the original Calypso system, but instead of being implanted, the radiofrequency beacon is placed on the patient's surface. It can be used anywhere on the body to track intra-fraction motion (such as respiration) in real time.

Answer 46

TomoTherapy uses a fan beam to image the patient prior to treatment. The 6 MV treatment beam is detuned to approximately 3.5 MV. Similar to a diagnostic CT, the fan beam is rotated around the patient while the treatment couch is translated through the machine. The exiting radiation is measured by a detector panel and reconstructed using filtered back-projection.

Yartsev S, Kron T, Van Dyk J. Tomotherapy as a tool in image-guided radiation therapy (IGRT): theoretical and technological aspects. *Biomedical Imaging and Interv J*. 2007;3(1):e16. doi:10.2349/biij.3.1.e16

Answer 47

The imaging dose is dependent on setting used during the scan, and patient anatomy, but it is normally 1 to 3 cGy. Since this dose is relatively low, it is suitable for daily use. It may also be accounted for in the treatment plan.

Answer 48

On a conventional linear accelerator, imaging is performed using a cone-shaped beam that rotates once around the patient. On a TomoTherapy machine, a fan-shaped beam is used for scanning the patient helically, as the couch and patient move through the gantry.

Question 49

In terms of scan time, how does a diagnostic CT-scanner compare to TomoTherapy's megavoltage computed tomography (MVCT), and to a cone beam computed tomography (CBCT) on a linear accelerator (linac)?

Question 50

What is a DRR?

Question 51

How is a digitally reconstructed radiograph (DRR) produced?

Question 52

What are the factors that affect the quality of a digitally reconstructed radiograph (DRR)?

Answer 49

A diagnostic CT-scanner, which can complete one rotation in a fraction of a second, is much faster than the MVCT on a TomoTherapy unit, which takes about 10 seconds per rotation. Newer CT-scanners also have a wider collimator, allowing them to image more of the patient in one rotation than TomoTherapy. A typical scan on the TomoTherapy unit can take 2 to 4 minutes depending on the extension of the patient scanned. This is longer than a CBCT scan on a linear accelerator, which takes around a minute, depending on gantry speed and arc length.

Answer 50

A DRR, or digitally reconstructed radiograph, is a computer-generated projection image produced from CT data. It shows a beam's-eye-view of the bony anatomy that can be compared to a portal image to check whether the patient is positioned as planned.

Answer 51

Using a virtual source position, ray lines are traced through the CT data to a virtual plane, at the distance of the imaging panel of the accelerator. The attenuation coefficients along each line are summed to produce an image at the virtual plane.

Answer 52

CT slice thickness, number of pixels, magnification of the DRR, and the step size are all factors that affect image quality.

Question 53

What equation is used to determine the attenuation along the ray lines used to construct a digitally reconstructed radiograph (DRR)?

Question 54

What is the Vision RT image-guidance system?

Question 55

When compared with other image-guided radiation therapy (IGRT) systems, what are some of Vision RT's advantages?

Question 56

Briefly describe ViewRay's MRIdian system.

Answer 53

$$\mu = \mu w\left(\frac{HU}{1,000}\right) + 1$$

where μ is the linear attenuation coefficient of tissue, μ_w is the linear attenuation coefficient of water, and HU is the Hounsfield unit.

Answer 54

Vision RTs main product is called AlignRT®. It is an optical surface-tracking system that uses two or three cameras, combined with a patterned-light projection, to visualize the surface of the patient's body. This image is compared to a reference surface image generated by the treatment planning system to make sure the patient surface is positioned correctly. It also provides real-time motion tracking, which can warn therapists of movements and can even switch off the radiation if movements exceed tolerances.

www.visionrt.com/products_solutions/alignrt

Answer 55

It can calculate source to skin distance (SSD) at any point on the patient during or after treatment, it allows users to define custom tolerances and will hold the beam automatically if they are exceeded, and it offers real-time monitoring and feedback. Additionally, internal fiducials or external markers on the skin are not necessary, and there is no imaging dose.

Answer 56

MRIdian is an MR-based radiation-therapy system. It uses MR imaging to visualize soft tissue and perform gated therapy in real time, without the use of implanted fiducials or other invasive procedures.

www.viewray.com/system

Question 57

How is radiation delivered with the ViewRay MRIdian?

Question 58

Many image-guided radiation therapy (IGRT) systems allow for real-time imaging. How is this useful?

Question 59

When using image-guided radiation therapy (IGRT), what is the difference between online and offline correction? Which is more common?

Answer 57

The MRIdian uses three heads loaded with cobalt-60 and spaced 120° apart. The three treatment heads can irradiate a patient simultaneously to improve delivery efficiency. The MRIdian produces the equivalent of a 4 MV linear accelerator (linac) beam. The system also uses three multileaf collimators for beam shaping and advanced treatments, such as intensity-modulated radiation therapy (IMRT).

Answer 58

Preimaging a patient, with cone beam computed tomography (CBCT), for example, is helpful to ensure correct positioning, but real-time imaging can ensure the patient is positioned correctly throughout treatment. It shows if any motion is occurring during treatment, and allows for beam holding if the target strays too far out of tolerance. By observing motion in real time, physicians can determine if margins are adequate.

Answer 59

An online correction strategy is when corrections are made before and during patient treatment. The information provided by image guidance is used to determine appropriate action. This accounts for both systematic and random errors. Offline correction is performed by analyzing several of the images from initial treatments and deciding on a strategy for future treatments. This method will not eliminate random error. Presently, online correction is more commonly used.

INDEX

Printed in the United States
By Bookmasters.

Printed in the United States
By Bookmasters